Measuring health

A review of quality of life measurement scales

Ann Bowling

Open University Press
Milton Keynes · Philadelphia

Open University Press
Celtic Court
22 Ballmoor
Buckingham
MK18 1XW

and
1900 Frost Road, Suite 101
Bristol, PA 19007, USA

First Published 1991. Reprinted 1992

British Library Cataloguing in Publication Data
Bowling, Ann
  Measuring health: a review of quality of life measurement
  scales.
  1. Health
  I. Title
  362.1042

  ISBN 0–335–15436–0
  ISBN 0–335–15435–2 (pbk)

Typeset by GCS, Leighton Buzzard, Beds.
Printed in Great Britain by Biddles Limited, Guildford and King's Lynn

Contents

Preface

The scales presented in this volume have been selected either because they have been well tested for reliability and validity, or because considerable interest has been expressed in their content area. Many of the broader measures of quality of life in relation to health status are relatively new and consequently underdeveloped and undertested.

While an attempt has been made to include the most popularly used and tested scales, omissions are inevitable in a volume of this size. The most notable omissions from this book are scales relating to specific diseases, for example, oncology and the numerous scales attempting to measure social stress and coping ability. Physicians have developed a number of scales which focus on problems specific to cancer patients (e.g. the Cancer Inventory of Problem Situations, by Schag *et al.* 1983); none have acceptable levels of reliability and validity and the area has been reviewed by Slevin *et al.* (1988). The measurement of stress and coping behaviour is also subject to tremendous debate which has not been resolved. Readers interested in these areas and their measurement issues should consult the comprehensive publications on this subject by Kasl and Cooper (1987) and Maes *et al.* (1987).

As some of the scales are only available commercially, it was not possible to obtain copyright permission to reproduce them in full in this volume. It was therefore decided to aim for consistency and to reproduce selected examples of all scales. Potential users are advised to consult the authors of scales before use in order to avoid copyright infringement. Informed use also assists authors of scales to compile bibliographies of users and results.

The reader will notice some variation in section length in the following chapters. This is simply because scales vary in length and also because some scales have been well tested and widely applied, while others have had more limited use. While it is not possible to present all applications of the scales contained here, each section contains a reasonable selection of the most pertinent publications. Section summaries have not been included advising readers on the 'best buy' as each scale presented has different advantages and disadvantages, and potential users need to consider these in relation to the aims and requirements of their research.

Acknowledgements

I would like to thank Jenny Stanley for her assistance in collating the many references consulted during the research for this book, and Dr Robert Edelmann for his helpful comments on the text.

List of abbreviations

ABS	Affect–Balance Scale
ADL	Index of Activities of Daily Living
AIMS	Arthritis Impact Measurement Scale
AMT	Abbreviated Mental Test
ASSIS	Arizona Social Support Interview Schedule
BDI	Beck Depression Inventory
CAPE	Clifton Assessment Procedures for the Elderly
CMI	Cornell Medical Index
CRBRS	Crichton Royal Behaviour Rating Scale
D–TFS	Delighted–Terrible Faces Scale
FAI	Functional Assessment Inventory
FRI	Family Relationship Index
GHQ	General Health Questionnaire
GMS	Geriatric Mental State
GWBS	(Psychological) General Well-Being Scale
HAD	Hospital Anxiety and Depression Scale
HAQ	Stanford Arthritis Center Health Assessment Questionnaire
HIS	Health Insurance Study
ISEL	Interpersonal Support Evaluation List
ISSB	Inventory of Socially Supportive Behaviours
ISSI	Interview Schedule for Social Interaction
LASA	Linear Analogue Self Assessment
LSIA	Life Satisfaction Index A
LSIB	Life Satisfaction Index B
LSIZ	Life Satisfaction Index Z
MHIQ	McMaster Health Index Questionnaire
MPQ	McGill Pain Questionnaire
MSQ	Mental Status Questionnaire

NHP	Nottingham Health Profile
OARS	Older American's Resource and Services Schedule
QL	Spitzer Quality of Life Index
QWBS	Quality of Well-Being Scale
SAD	Symptoms of Anxiety and Depression Scale
SIP	Sickness Impact Profile
SNS	Social Network Scale
SS-A	Social Support Appraisals Scale
SS-B	Social Support Behaviours Scale
UCLA	University of California at Los Angeles
WHO	World Health Organization

1
The conceptualization of functioning, health and quality of life

Clinicians and researchers interested in health care are increasingly focusing their attention on the measurement of health outcomes, or consequences, of care. The conceptualization and measurement of outcomes are controversial. There is now recognition that meaningful measures of health-related quality of life should be used to evaluate health-care interventions. Most existing indicators reflect a 'disease' model. The 'disease' model is a medical conception of pathological abnormality which is indicated by a set of signs and symptoms. A person's 'ill health' is indicated by feelings of pain and discomfort or perceptions of change in usual functioning and feeling. Illnesses can be the result of pathological abnormality, but not necessarily so. A person can feel ill without medical science being able to detect disease. Measures of health status need to take both concepts into account. What matters in the 20th century is how the patient feels, rather than how doctors think they ought to feel on the basis of clinical measurements. Symptom response or survival rates are no longer enough; and, particularly where people are treated for chronic or life-threatening conditions, the therapy has to be evaluated in terms of whether it is more or less likely to lead to an outcome of a life worth living in social and psychological, as well as physical, terms.

Measuring health outcome

In order to measure health outcome a measure of health status is required which in turn must be based on a concept of health. The limitations of the widely used negative definition of health as the absence of disease and the World Health Organization's (WHO) 1946 definition of health as total social, psychological and physical well-being have long been recognized (WHO 1958). In the absence of satisfactory definitions of this basic concept how should health outcome be defined? Typical indices of health status in current use in the Western world focus on disease, illness and negative concepts. They include mortality rates and biochemical data (e.g. haemoglobin levels); routinely collected statistics on health-service use; subjective indicators: self- or other-reported morbidity, disability and behavioural data (e.g. smoking, alcohol use, etc.).

Mortality and morbidity indicators used by clinicians

Clinicians ultimately tend to judge the value of a therapy in terms of the five-year-survival period. In the developed world mortality rates are routinely collected; on the other hand, mortality statistics are subject to error and also ignore the living – many health-care programmes and interventions will have little or no impact on mortality rates. Survival time needs to be interpreted more broadly in terms of the impact and consequences of treatment.

The major outcome measures in most clinical trials are mortality and morbidity. Measures of morbidity used by clinicians in assessing outcome commonly focus on results of biochemical tests, observed symptom rates or role performance (e.g. number of days off work, bed disability days). Wilson Barnett (1981) has reviewed research attempting to measure outcome among post-operative cardiac patients. She reported that the most frequently used measures related to mortality rates (length of survival), morbidity (serious complication), physical condition (e.g. exercise testing, cardiac function, angiography), patency of grafts, symptoms (pain, dyspnoea) and return to work. Return to work is one of the most commonly used non-biological indicators of health status. This is of limited value as it is influenced by economic and social opportunities and age.

Service utilization

Another source of data to which there is relatively easy access in the USA and the UK in particular is service-use information. The USA relies heavily on health insurance data for information about service use, the UK relies on routinely collected information from the National Health Service about deaths and discharges from hospital by condition, age and sex. Some information is also available from periodic morbidity surveys in general medical practice. Much of Europe has little tradition of data collection of this type. All routinely collected data about usage is subject to problems of inaccuracy. Also, while hospital readmission rates, length of hospital stay and other indices of service use are frequently used as outcome and morbidity measures, they often reflect the policies of individual clinicians and service provision, and provide no information about the impact of the treatment on the patient's life.

Subjective health indicators

More detailed information about health and illness is only available from surveys. These take the form of either community-based population surveys, which collect data about individuals' self-reports of illness and disability, or studies of clinic populations based on patient-, and sometimes physician-assessed, morbidity.

An example of a physician-assessed morbidity-rating scale is the Olsson Health Scale which was developed using New York Heart Association gradings which range from 'dead' to 'alive' with various complications, to 'alive' with I to IV grades of activity limitation (Olsson *et al.* 1986). The classifications give no indication of the effects of the condition on specific areas of physical, economic, psychological, social and domestic functioning. This also provides an example of how, in relation to the assessment of morbidity, health is generally conceptualized as being at one extreme of a continuum, generally defined negatively as the absence of symptoms, and with death at the other. There are differing views as to the gradations that may exist between 'perfect health' and 'death'. For example, Dorn (1955) represents the health spectrum as perfect health at one end, passing through conditions predisposing to disease (e.g. obesity), latent or incipient disease, early apparent disease, far advanced disease and then to death. The problem with such frameworks is that each stage is blurred as a disease may or may not manifest itself for a period of time and may or may not be recognized by the individual or presented to, and diagnosed by, a doctor. Moreover, in passing along the continuum, the point at which a state of health no longer exists is unknown.

A more positive model is a scale of feeling, or well-being. Merrell and Reed (1949) proposed a graded scale of health from positive to negative health:

> On such a scale people would be classified from those who are in top-notch condition with abundant energy, through to people who are well, to fairly well, down to people who are feeling rather poorly, and finally to the definitely ill. The word health rather than illness is chosen deliberately to emphasise the positive side of this scale, for in the past we have focussed our attention thoroughly on the disease side.

The authors criticize scales which range from 'no reported illness' to 'hospitalization' or 'confinement to bed' as they do not break down the title 'no reported illness' into different degrees of positive health and well-being. Classifications along continuums, whether negative or positive in orientation, appear relatively crude. They are reflective of the underdeveloped state of measures of health outcome.

Routine information about illness, obtained from individuals responding to large community samples, has been collected annually by government interview surveys in the USA, since 1956, in the UK since 1971, and in Finland since 1964. There is also an increasing number of *ad hoc* surveys carried out by research organizations, university and health departments.

Routine government health surveys typically report on the incidence of acute illness and injuries requiring either medical attention or restriction of daily activity; number of days of restricted activity and activity limitation resulting from various diseases and conditions; absence from work or school; self-reported chronic diseases and impairments; and discharges from hospital. Some also include symptom check-lists. Early methodologies concentrated on the collection of morbidity data, reflecting a disease model. More recent studies also reflect this model but are also more likely to encompass a behavioural approach – e.g. the annual UK General Household Survey often includes questions on behaviour such as alcohol and tobacco use.

There are multiple influences upon patient outcome, and these require a broad model of health. The non-biological factors which can affect recovery and outcome include patient psychology, motivation and adherence to therapy, socioeconomic status, availability of health care, social support networks and individual and cultural beliefs and behaviours. Outcome should thus also be measured more comprehensively in relation to people's value systems. More recently developed 'subjective health indicators' reflect these non-biological inputs. They are also recognized in research on health behaviour, for example the health-belief model refers to people's perceptions of the severity of an illness, their susceptibility to it, and the costs and benefits incurred in following a particular course of action (Becker 1974).

Health status has been operationalized in most survey and broader clinical-outcomes research in terms of self-reported health-status and, perhaps most commonly, by functional ability. The following sections examine the concepts of functional ability and status, followed by the broader concepts of positive health, social health, and quality of life.

The concept of functional ability

One of the most common methods of assessing outcome of care in a broader sense is in terms of people's ability to perform tasks of daily living. Disability measures are more meaningful to people's lives than objective biochemical measures or measures of timed walking or grip strength.

The terms 'impairment', 'disability' and 'handicap' are often erroneously used interchangeably. The increasing use of the concept of functional dependency has recently added to the confusion. The distinctions between these concepts first requires clarification. The World Health Organization's (1980) 'International Classification of Impairments, Disabilities and Handicaps' provides a consistent terminology and a classification system.

This defines the terms 'impairment', 'disability' and 'handicap' and links them together conceptually:

Disease or ⎯⎯⎯▶ Impairment ⎯⎯▶ Disability ⎯⎯⎯▶ Handicap
Disorder

e.g.:

Blindness ⎯⎯⎯▶ Vision ⎯⎯⎯▶ Seeing ⎯⎯⎯▶ Orientation

Rheumatism ⎯⎯▶ Skeletal ⎯⎯⎯▶ Walking ⎯⎯▶ Mobility

Impairment is defined as: 'In the context of health experience, an impairment is any loss or abnormality of psychological, physiological or anatomical structure or function.' It represents deviation from some norm in the individual's biomedical status. While impairment is concerned with biological function, disability is concerned with activities expected of the person or the body.

Disability is defined as 'In the context of health experience, a disability is any restriction or lack (resulting from an impairment) of ability to perform an activity in the manner or within the range considered normal for a human being.'

Functional handicap represents the social consequences of impairments or disabilities. It is thus a social phenomenon and a relative concept. The attitudes and values of the non-handicapped play a major part in defining a handicap. It is defined as:

In the context of health experience, a handicap is a disadvantage for a given individual, resulting from an impairment or a disability, that limits or prevents the fulfilment of a role that is normal (depending on age, sex and social and cultural factors) for that individual.

These constitute working definitions of impairment, disability and handicap. A working definition, as distinct from an operational definition, must be precise enough to suggest the content of the indicators but must not be so precise that it cannot be generalized to a variety of contexts. Operational definitions, in contrast, are usually specific to a particular measurement instrument and even to a particular type of study. They define the specific behaviours and the ways in which they are to be classified.

These concepts lead to the concept of dependency on other people or service providers. Impairment and disability may or may not lead to dependency in the same way they lead to handicap. As with the concept of handicap, functional 'dependency' is a social consequence – societal attitudes decide on its definition and existence. Wilkin (1987) defined dependency as 'A state in which an individual is reliant upon other(s) for assistance in meeting recognized needs.'

In summary, impairment and disability may lead to dependency in the same way they lead to handicap. However, they cannot be equated with dependency, nor is there a necessary relationship.

Working definitions are limited to specific contexts which, in the case of dependency, means that they tend to deal with particular types of dependency, for example, the type of help necessary for survival that has to be obtained from others.

Operational definitions, on the whole, concentrate upon activities of daily living, often sub-divided into domestic and self-care activities. Thus the operational definition of dependency is failure to perform certain specified activities independently to a pre-defined standard.

Functional status

On the basis of the previous definitions, functional status can be defined as the degree to which an individual is able to perform socially allocated roles free of physically (or mentally in the case of mental illness) related limitations.

There is a clear distinction from general health status. Functional status is directly related to the ability to perform social roles, which a measure of general health need not take into account. Functional status is just one component of health – it is a measure of the effects of disease rather than the disease itself.

The concept of positive health

Health is usually referred to negatively as the absence of disease, illness and sickness. All measures of health status take health as a baseline and then measure deviations away from this. They are really measuring ill health. It is easier to measure departures from health rather than to find indices of health itself. When studying severely ill populations, the best strategy may be to employ measures of negative health status. However, only approximately 15 per cent of a general population in a Western society will have chronic physical limitations, and some 10–20 per cent will have substantial psychiatric impairment (Stewart et al. 1978; Ware et al. 1979). Thus reliance on a negative definition of health provides little information about the health of the remaining 80–90 per cent of general populations. A positive conception of health is difficult to measure because of the lack of agreement over its definition. Clinical judgements focus upon the absence of disease; lay people may hold a variety of concepts such as the ability to carry out normal everyday tasks, feeling strong, good, fit and so on. Without an operational definition it is not possible to determine if and when a state of health has been achieved by a population.

The WHO has recommended the development of measures of positive health (Scottish Health Education Group 1984). In its 1946 constitution (WHO 1958), the WHO specified that 'Health is a state of complete physical, mental and social wellbeing and not merely the absence of disease and infirmity.' No conceptual or operational definitions were provided. Despite the controversy provoked by this utopian definition, it has generated a new focus on a broader, more positive concept of health, rather than a narrow, negative (disease-based) focus (Seedhouse 1986). The World Health Organization's (1985) ideal of 'Health for all by the Year 2000' and the *Ottawa Charter for Health Promotion* (1986) with its emphasis on assisting the individual to increase control over and improve health, both employ broader definitions of health than those traditionally employed. They highlight the inadequacy of existing negative concepts of health (Thuriaux 1988).

There is now broad agreement that the concept of positive health is more than the mere absence of disease or disability and implies 'completeness' and 'full functioning' or 'efficiency' of mind and body and social adjustment. Beyond this there is no one accepted definition. Positive health could be described as the ability to cope with stressful situations, the maintenance of a strong social-support system, integration in the community, high morale and life satisfaction, psychological well-being, and even levels of physical fitness as well as physical health (Lamb, *et al.* 1988). It is composed of distinct components that must be measured and interpreted separately.

Partly confusing conceptual issues further are the other related multi-faceted concepts such as 'social well-being' or 'social health' and 'quality of life', which are components of a broad concept of positive health.

The concept of social health

Donald *et al.* (1978) have called a broader view of health than the reporting of symptoms, illness and functional ability 'social health'. Social health was viewed as a dimension of individual well-being distinct from both physical and mental health. They conceptualized social health both as a component of health-status outcomes (as a dependent variable) and, following Caplan (1974) and Cassell (1976):

> in terms of social support systems that might intervene and modify the effect of the environment and life stress events on physical and mental health (as an intervening variable). Measurement of social

health focuses on the individual and is defined in terms of inter-personal interactions (e.g. visits with friends) and social participation (e.g. membership in clubs). Both objective and subjective constructs (e.g. number of friends and a rating of how well one is getting along, respectively) are included in this definition.

(Donald *et al.* 1978).

The authors attempted to measure social health, or social well-being as they also sometimes called it, in the Rand health insurance study.

Other authors have also conceptualized social health as a separate component of health status, defining it in terms of the degree to which people function adequately as members of the community (Renne 1974; Greenblatt 1975). Lerner (1973) noted that health status may be a function of non-health factors external to the individual, such as the environment, the community and significant social groups. He recommended that social well-being measures focus on constructs such as role-related coping, family health and social participation. He hypothesized that socially healthy persons would be more able to cope successfully with day-to-day challenges arising from performance of major social roles; would live in families that are more stable, integrated and cohesive; would be more likely to participate in community activities; and would be more likely to conform to societal norms. In relation to psychiatric illness, Leighton (1959) has described how individual personalities can be influenced by the quality and quantity of interpersonal relationships. Lack of social integration may produce psychological stress and decrease the individual's resources for dealing with it, possibly resulting in psychiatric disorders. Lack of social support has also been implicated in poor outcome of depressive illness (George *et al.* 1989).

Social support can thus be regarded as a key concept in theory and research on 'social health'. Kaplan (1975) outlined several areas of social support, including work achievements and position in the hierarchy; family support, social activity and friendships; financial adequacy; personal life (e.g. existence of a confidante); personal achievements and philosophy and sexual satisfaction. In sum, studies of social health tend to focus on the individual, rather than on the community and the concept is used as a dimension of another imprecisely defined term: 'quality of life'.

The concept of quality of life

In general terms quality can be defined as a grade of 'goodness'. Quality of life is a broader concept than personal health status and also takes social well-being, as described above, into account. There is no consensus over a definition of quality of life. The literature covers a range of components: functional ability including role functioning (e.g. domestic, return to work), the degree and quality of social and community interaction, psychological well-being, somatic sensation (e.g. pain) and life satisfaction. It is becoming fashionable to equate all non-clinical data with 'quality of life' which is likely to be a source of conceptual confusion. Health and functional status are just two dimensions of health-related quality of life.

There is little empirical research attempting to define those qualities which make life and survival valuable. Mendola and Pelligrini (1979) have defined quality of life as 'the individual's achievement of a satisfactory social situation within the limits of perceived physical capacity'. This is a fairly limited definition and no more easy to operationalize than more complex definitions. Shin and Johnson (1978) have suggested that quality of life consists of 'the possession of resources necessary to the satisfaction of individual needs, wants and desires, participation in activities enabling personal development and self actualization and satisfactory comparison between oneself and others', all of which are dependent on previous experience and knowledge. Patterson (1975) approached this differently by identifying certain characteristics deemed essential to any evaluation of quality of life. These included general health, performance status, general comfort, emotional status and economic status, all of which are contributory to the proposition made by Shin and Johnson. Basically quality of life is recognized as a concept representing individual responses to the physical, mental and social effects of illness on daily living which influence the extent to which personal satisfaction with life circumstances can be achieved. It encompasses more than adequate physical well-being, it includes perceptions of well-being, a basic level of satisfaction and a general sense of self-worth. It is an abstract and complex concept comprising diverse areas, all of which contribute to the whole, personal satisfaction and self-esteem.

Studies of quality of life after various therapies have been reviewed by several authors. They have consistently reached the same conclusion that most studies of quality of life are hampered by poor design and inadequate assessment methods. Reviews of clinical trials of treatment also report that elements of quality of life were mentioned in between 3–50 per cent of studies and measured in fewer than 2–7 per cent (Bardelli and Saracci 1978; McPeek and McPeek 1984; O'Young and McPeek 1987).

Wilson Barnett (1981) in her review of studies of recovery after cardiac surgery reported that measures purporting to tap quality of life in a social and psychological sense were rarely used. Rarely used measures included activity levels (other than work), compliance with medical advice, social activities (hobbies), financial status, sexual activity and patient satisfaction with the operation. Exceptionally, evaluation criteria used to assess outcome included psychological status (affect, adjustment, self-esteem, perception of health status), resumption of normal life, 'minor' physical problems, patient satisfaction with advice and guidance, and patient understanding of treatment. She concluded that the implication is that more social and psychological measures are needed.

Quality of life as an outcome measure: whose assessment?

Existing global measurement scales of health outcome, aiming to encompass the measurement of 'quality of life' are based on either physicians' or individuals' own assessments.

The question arises about who should measure quality of life. McNeil *et al.*'s (1978; 1981) research shows that doctors, nurses, medical students, volunteers and patients disagree over treatment of choice for lung cancer and cancer of the larynx. Research indicates wide discrepancies between patients' and doctors' ratings of outcome after specific therapies (Orth-Gomer *et al.* 1979; Thomas and Lyttle 1980; Jachuck *et al.* 1982).

Slevin *et al.* (1988) attempted to determine whether assessments of quality of life of cancer patients by health professionals are meaningful and reliable by analysing the associations between professionals' and patients' assessments. The instruments used were the Karnofsky Performance Scale, the Spitzer Quality of Life Index, the Hospital Anxiety and Depression Scale and a series of linear analogue self-assessment scales. The wide discrepancies between doctors' and patients' assessments led the authors to conclude that doctors could not adequately measure the patients' quality of life. The implication is that measures of outcome should take account of individuals' self-assessments. While a number of self-rating scales exist and will be reviewed in the following chapters, few indicators attempt to measure patients' perceptions of improvement or satisfaction with level of performance; yet it is this element which is largely responsible for predicting whether individuals seek care, accept treatment and consider themselves to be well and 'recovered'.

Measures of health status in relation to quality of life

Developments in measures of health status have been largely confined to the USA and the UK. A recent evaluation of the 32 European member states of the WHO (Thuriaux 1988) reported that attempts at quantitative measurement of health status were only mentioned in two countries; and data on the measurement of freedom from disability such as independence in activities of daily living, the proportion of disabled people in employment or measures of temporary or long-term disability, were provided by only five member states. Information generally available was largely limited to indicators such as overall tobacco and cigarette consumption from trade sources, and proportions of low-birthweight babies.

Whilst a plethora of quantitative tools exist which operationalize and attempt to measure aspects of quality of life which are regarded as pertinent to health status, such as life satisfaction, well-being and morale, functional ability, social interaction, stress and psychiatric disturbance, attempts to combine them into a single tool have been less successful. Most of these attempts have been made in the USA, generally producing diverse, unwieldy and time-consuming scales of measurement. Moreover, the conceptual confusion which surrounds definitions of health in relation to quality of life is reflected in these measurement tools.

During the 1980s, as a result of the increasing focus on health promotion, the search for indicators of positive health has intensified and has again been stimulated by the WHO (Abelin *et al.* 1986; Anderson *et al.* 1989). The WHO's concept of health in social, psychological and physical terms has become accepted to the extent that a measure of health status that fails to incorporate one of these dimensions is subject to negative evaluation (Kaplan 1985). Attempts have been made to measure well-being. One example is the McMaster Health Index Questionnaire (Chambers 1982) which includes questions on general well-being. An index of psychological well-being was developed by Bradburn (1969) and a similar one by Dupuy (1984). These types of scales are gradually being incorporated into studies of health-related quality of life. Progress is sometimes slow due to the differences of opinion between researchers and policy makers with regard to the definition and measurement of health. Researchers are increasingly inclining towards self-ratings of present health; personal evaluation of physical condition; feelings of anxiety, nerves, depression; feelings of general positive affect; and future expectations about health. On the other hand, policy makers may prefer more explicit indicators in their formation of health policy: limitations in activities of daily living; confinement to bed due to ill health; ratings of intensity, duration and frequency of pain (Noack and McQueen 1988).

Whatever perspective is adopted, the reliability and validity of existing measures are still questionable, especially as most are derived from professional conceptions of well-being. Two measures which were derived from interviews with lay people are the Sickness Impact Profile and the Nottingham Health Profile, but these both limited respondents to assessing the effects of illness on behaviour, rather than global conceptualizations of health-related quality of life. The range of available health indicators consists of *ad hoc* measures that may or may not focus on functioning and health related behaviours, morbidity and perceived health. Many of these measures have serious limitations in terms of reliability, validity and techniques of analysis, although attempts are continuing to refine and develop the most popular scales.

2
Theory of measurement

Choice of health indicator

When deciding on which measure to use, the investigator should assess whether a disease-specific or broad-ranging instrument is required; the type of scoring that the instrument is based on (whether scores can be easily analysed in relation to other variables); the reliability, validity and sensitivity of the scale; the appropriateness of the instrument for the study population; the acceptability of the instrument to the group under study (Hunt *et al.* 1986). It is also important to decide whether the study requires measurement on a nominal-, ordinal-, interval- or ratio-scale level; these terms are explained below.

Measurement theory

Descriptions can be placed on a nominal or an ordinal, interval or ratio scale. The requisite level of measurement depends on the intended applications of the indicator and on the question the researcher is attempting to answer.

With a *nominal* scale, numbers or other symbols are used simply to classify a characteristic or item. This is measurement at its weakest level. For example, functional disability states and perceived health are defined by descriptions and thus a nominal or classification scale is constructed. For the purpose of the comparative evaluation of the outcome of intervention A in comparison with the outcome of intervention B a nominal scale may be sufficient (for example, 'died' or 'survived').

Hypotheses can be tested regarding the distribution of cases among categories by using the nonparametric test, x^2, and also Fisher's exact probability test. The most common measure of association (correlation) for nominal data is the contingency coefficient.

An *ordinal* (or ranking) scale is applicable where objects in one category of a scale are not simply different from objects in other categories of that scale, but they stand in some kind of relation to them. For example, typical relations may be higher than, more preferred, more difficult (in effect, greater than). This is an ordinal scale. Many disability and health-status measures are strictly of this type.

The most appropriate statistic for describing the central tendency of scores in an ordinal scale is the median, since the median is not affected by changes of any scores above or below it as long as the number of scores above and below remain the same. Hypotheses can be tested using nonparametric statistics such as correlation coefficients based on rankings (e.g. Spearman r or the Kendall r). An ordinal scale is sufficient only for answering basic questions such as 'How does X compare with Y?'

An *interval* scale is obtained when a scale has all the characteristics of an ordinal scale, and when in addition the distances between any two numbers on the scale are of known size. Measurement considerably stronger than ordinality has thus been achieved. An interval scale is characterized by a common and constant unit of measurement which assigns a real number, but the zero point and unit of measurement are arbitrary (e.g. temperature – two scales are commonly used as the zero point differs on each and is arbitrary).

The interval scale is a truly quantitative scale and all the common parametric statistics (means, standard deviations, Pearson correlations, etc.) are applicable as are the common statistical tests of significance (t test, F test, etc.). Parametric tests should be used as nonparametric methods would not usually take advantage of all information contained in the research data. Interval scales are appropriate if the question is 'How different is X to Y?'

The *ratio* scale exists when a scale has all the characteristics of an interval scale and in addition has a true zero point as its origin. The ratio of any two scale points is independent of the unit of measurement. Weight is one example. Any statistical test is usable when ratio measurement has been achieved. Ratio scales are needed if the question is: 'Proportionately how different is X to Y?'

The most rigorous methods of data analysis require quantitative data. Whenever possible, measures which yield interval or ratio data should be used, although this is often difficult in social science. Measures of functional disability and health status never strictly reach a ratio- or interval-scale of measurement. However, methods of data transformation do exist which permit even nominal data to be made quantitative for purposes of analysis.

Measurement problems

Measurement problems are rife when attempting measures of health outcomes. Indicators may work well or badly and are usually assessed by tests of validity and reliability.

Authors of the various measures often make claims for reliability and validity based on achieved coefficients without any reference to acceptable levels. Suggestions for acceptable levels for reliability and validity range from 0.85 to 0.94, although often 0.50 is regarded as acceptable for correlation coefficients (Ware *et al.* 1980). A full discussion of the problems of achieving reliability and validity can be found in Streiner and Norman (1989).

Validity

Validity is concerned with whether the indicator actually does measure the underlying attribute or not. One of the most problematic aspects of assessing validity is the varying terminology. Textbooks have tended to focus on content validity, criterion validity and construct validity. More recently, more different types of validity have emerged. Construct validity has been differentiated into various dimensions such as discriminant validity and convergent validity. However, all types of validity are addressing the same issue of the degree of confidence that can be placed on the inferences drawn from scale scores. These issues have been addressed more fully by Messick (1980) and Streiner and Norman (1989).

The assessment of validity involves assessment against a standard criterion. Because there is no 'gold standard' of health against which health-status indices can be compared, the validation methods commonly used in the behavioural sciences are the assessment of content and construct validity (American Psychological Association 1974). The criteria of validity which should be met in general are:

Content validity
Do the components of the scale/item cover *all* aspects of the attribute to be measured? Does the content of the variable match the name which it has been given? Each item should fall into at least one of the content areas being tapped. If it does not, then the item is not relevant to the scale's objectives, or the list of scale objectives is not comprehensive. The number of items in each area should also reflect its importance to the attribute.

Face validity
This is one form of content validity. Is the indicator, on the face of it, a reasonable one – do the items appear to be measuring the variables they claim to measure? Is the meaning and relevance of the indicator self-evident?

Criterion validity
Can the variable be measured with accuracy? The traditional definition of criterion validity is the correlation of a scale with some other measure of the trait under study, ideally a 'gold standard'. Criterion validity is usually divided into two types: concurrent and predictive validity:

Concurrent validity   This refers to a scale's substitutability and involves the correlation of the new scale with the criterion measure; both scales are administered to subjects at the same time. It is most often used when attempting to develop a replacement scale which is simpler or less expensive to administer than an existing scale.

Predictive validity   Does the measure predict future differences? With predictive validity, the criterion will be unavailable until some future end point.

Construct validity
This type of validity is relevant in more abstract areas such as psychology and sociology where the variable of interest cannot be directly observed. Underlying psychological or sociological factors are referred to as hypothetical constructs. These are the theories which attempt to explain behaviours and attitudes. There is no one single study that can satisfy the criteria for establishing construct validity (or testing constructs), it is an ongoing process. There are many predictions that could be made from one construct. Unlike other types of validity testing, testing for construct validity involves assessing both theory and method simultaneously. The problem is that, if the predictions made on the basis of theory are not confirmed, then the problem could be with the validity of the measure or the validity of the theory. This type of validity is generally divided into convergent and discriminant validity:

Convergent–Discriminant validity   This involves assessing the extent to which the new scale is related to other variables and measures of the same construct to which it should be related. For example, if the theory states that depressed subjects will perceive their level of social support to be lower than non-depressed people, then the scores from scales measuring these two dimensions should be correlated. The interpretation is sometimes problematic with the measurement of similar concepts, as scale scores that correlate too highly may be measuring the same dimension.Convergent validity also requires that a new scale should correlate with other measures of this construct. Thus, while convergent validity requires correlation with related variables, discriminant validity requires that the construct should not correlate with dissimilar variables.

Factor analysis is an increasingly used technique for the assessment of the number of dimensions that underlie a set of variables. If items relate to a single dimension, then the combination of items into a single measure is supported. If the items relate to a number of different dimensions, then refinement of the scale or sub-scale analyses are more appropriate in recognition of this (Harman 1976).

Reliability

An instrument will also require testing for reliability. A measure is judged to be reliable when it consistently produces the same results, particularly when applied to the same subjects at different time periods. Three methods of measuring reliability are commonly used – multiple form, split half and test-retest. In addition, tests of internal consistency based on statistical models, for example using factor analysis are becoming more widespread (Harman 1976).

Multiple form reliability
This is used where two instruments, which have been developed in parallel, and which measure the same attribute, are administered and the scores on each correlated. A high correlation indicates a reliable test.

Split-half reliability
This is a method of assessing internal consistency where items on an instrument are divided into two equivalent parts and correlations between the scores on each part are computed. This requires that the items in the instrument should be homogeneous with respect to the attribute being measured. This is useful when a large pool of items measures one attribute.

Test-retest reliability
The test is administered to the same population on two occasions and the results are compared, usually by correlation. The main problem with this is that the first administration may affect responses on the second. There can be problems with interpretation of observed change, given the potential for observer errors with any scale, and the potential for genuine individual change between administration which affects the estimate of reliability.

   The achievement of standards of validity and reliability requires time and effort. It is a powerful reason for using existing scales.

Types of survey instruments

Most instruments used in social science rely on self-reporting of feelings, attitudes and behaviour by people in an interview situation or in response to a self-administered questionnaire. Other measurement approaches include the use of records and the observation of behaviour. Each approach has its strengths and limitations. The optimal measurement strategy is to measure the same phenomenon using several different approaches (Webb *et al.* 1966).

Self-report measures

Self-report measures are essential for much research because of the need to obtain subjective assessments of experiences (e.g. feelings about recovery, level of health and well-being). They have a broad appeal as they are often quick to administer and involve little interpretation by the investigator. Self-report measures may take a variety of forms:

Single-item measures   These are self-report questions which use a single question, rating or item to measure the concept of interest.

Battery   A series of self-report questions, ratings or items used to measure a concept. The responses are not summed or weighted. A battery is like a series of single item measures, all tapping the same concept.

Scale   A series of self-report questions, ratings or items used to measure a concept. The response categories of the items are all in the same format, are summed and may be weighted.

Sometimes researchers do not wish to use a long scale, because their questionnaires are already fairly lengthy, and prefer single-item questions. Generally, where questionnaire length permits, scales are preferred because they contain a larger number of items and are suitable for statistical calculations using summed and weighted scores. Single-item measures are least preferable because it is doubtful that one question can effectively tap a given phenomenon and it is also difficult to assess the adequacy of a single-item instrument.

Scaling item responses

There is a wide variety of scaling methods for item responses. The finer the distinctions that can be made between subjects' responses, the greater the precision of the measure. For example, rather than asking a person to simply agree or disagree with a statement (which yields only two-response (nominal) categories), it is preferable to ask respondents to indicate their opinions along a continuum of agreement: e.g. 'strongly disagree, disagree, no opinion, agree or strongly agree' (Likert 1952). Attitudinal and behavioural issues are not easily dichotomized; they often lie on a continuum. A question about any difficulty in washing oneself can elicit a range of responses from 'no difficulty', to 'slight', 'moderate' or 'severe' difficulty, to 'cannot do this at all'. Offering a wide range of choices is likely to reduce the potential for error due to confusion, although the continuum should not be too great, or meaningless responses will be elicited.

. If the aim of the research is to elicit continuous rather than categorical responses, there are several techniques available. One approach is to ask respondents to indicate their replies on a visual analogue scale – for example, a line of 100 mm, with descriptions such as 'very depressed' to 'not at all depressed' at each end. Respondents are asked to place a mark on the line corresponding to their state. Another method is to offer respondents a choice of discrete responses: 'Would you describe your health for your age as excellent, good, fair or poor?'

Another well-known example is Thurstone's method. This involves asking respondents to rank statements relating to the variable of interest, which are typed onto cards, into hierarchical order, from the most to the least desirable. The details and scoring systems of this technique are described by Streiner and Norman (1989) and in most psychology and methodology textbooks.

In relation to functional status, many methods exist of scoring or assessing 'function' by scaling, whereby a set of items can be put in a hierarchy of severity. The notion is that patients who can perform a particular task will be able to perform all tasks more easily. Conversely, if they cannot perform a particular task, they will be unable to perform tasks rated as higher. Guttman's (1944) scaling of disability was one of the earliest attempts in this field. He ranked degrees of patient disability in respect of a number of activities, such as feeding, continence, ambulation, dressing and bathing. This method assumes that disabilities can be ordered. Provided that disability progressed steadily from one activity to another (i.e. patients first have difficulty in bathing, then in bathing and dressing, and so on until they are disabled in respect of all five activities), this method of scaling yields a single rating from 1 (no disability) to 6 (disabled on all five). For example, four disabilities always score worse than three, and a score of 6 would assume that all disability items 2–5 had been affirmed. Examples of well-known measures using this scaling method are the Index of Activities of Daily Living (ADL) and the Arthritis Impact Measurement Scale (AIMS). A more recent Guttman scaling instrument has been developed by Williams et al. (1976). The activities which make up the scale are not comprehensive in terms of describing activities of daily living. The instrument has the advantage of having two scales, one for men and one for women. Work on developing and refining the scale is continuing. Guttman scaling, although popular, has been criticized for its method of attributing equal weights to item responses. For example, with responses per item ranging from 1 to 6, the higher the score the greater the debility; it cannot be assumed that 6 is six times as bad as 1 (Skinner and Yett 1972).

Weighting scale items

Many scales simply involve summing the item scores, each of which has been given an equal weight. This is the easiest solution to the scale scoring. There is a fundamental problem with this method: some items may be more important to the construct underlying the scale than others and should therefore contribute more to the total score. Summing also erroneously converts what is at best ordinal data into interval levels of measurement when applying statistical techniques. Statistical caution is required.

The problem with many scoring methods, particularly when equal weight for each item is applied, is that a given score can be arrived at in different ways. A person who is cheerful and lucid but unable to walk due to arthritis may achieve the same scale score as someone who is physically mobile but disoriented and withdrawn. While this may be useful for assessments of staff workload, it is not useful in assessing patient outcome in any detail. Scoring may exacerbate the instrument's distortion of the experiences of individuals. The problem may be avoided by treating all aspects of disability and health status as equal contributors to overall severity, and expressing the results for each item separately. The disadvantage of this method is that multiple disabilities are not then evidence and this type of breakdown can be cumbersome in analysis. The alternative is to assign different values (weights) to different scale items for scoring purposes. The Normative Scale relies on the classification of items into major or minor categories, e.g. with disability items, 'being able to feed oneself' is given twice the weight of 'being able to dress oneself'. Principle Component Scaling relies on the internal evidence of the data being scaled, thus calculating the relative weights to be given to each item to construct a linear additive index. Numerous health-index questionnaires fall into these categories. The main methods of weighting have been clearly and fully described by Streiner and Norman (1989). The most common is to use a different number of items to measure the various aspects of the trait, proportional to its importance within the construct. The total for any sub-scale would be the number of items with a response of interest divided by the total number of items within the sub-scale. The sub-scale scores can be added together for the scale total. Thus, each sub-scale contributes equally to the scale's total score, even though each may consist of a different number of items.

In practice, however, it is frequently found that weighting items makes little difference to subjects' relative scores, despite the inherent logic of this technique. This is because people who score high on one scale variant often score high on others. Examples of this have been given by Streiner and Norman (1989). On the other hand, weighting items can increase the predictive ability of an index (Perloff and Persons 1988). Streiner and Norman (1989) conclude that when the scale contains at least 40 items, or when the items are fairly homogeneous, then differential weighting contributes little (except complexity in scoring).

Utility rating scales

Finally, economists have devised a series of econometric scaling techniques in an attempt to assign a numerical value to a health state. These are known as utility ratings, the most well-known application of these being the quality-adjusted life year (Chiange 1965; Rosser and Watts 1971; Kaplan and Bush 1982). These will be only briefly referred to here; interested readers should consult specialist texts for their evaluation (e.g. Torrance 1986; Teeling Smith 1988).

The rating scale

The rating scale is suitable for measuring preferences for chronic or temporary health states. A typical rating scale consists of a line drawn on a page with clearly defined end points such as 'death/least desirable' at one end and 'healthy/most desirable' at the other. The remaining health states are then located on the line between these two in order of their preference, such that the intervals between them correspond to the differences in preference between the health states, as perceived by the subject. This is the interval-scaling technique. The scale is measured from 0 assigned to the worst health state of the group and 1 assigned to the best. The subject is asked to select the best and worst health states from the group and then locate the other states on the scale relative to each other, according to the interval-scaling principle.

The standard gamble

With this technique, subjects are asked to choose between a gamble, with a desirable outcome, with risk P, and a less desirable outcome, with risk 1-P, and a certain option of intermediate desirability. The subject is asked what probability of getting the desirable or less desirable outcome will make him indifferent between the gamble and the certainty.

An example of the standard gamble is to take a person faced with the choice of remaining in a poor state of health versus taking a gamble on treatment that could fully restore health or result in death (e.g. surgery for angina). If the probability of restoring full health is varied there will be a point where the person is indifferent between her current poor state of health and taking the gamble of surgery. If the person perceives her poor health state as particularly undesirable, she will be more likely to accept a greater probability of death in order to escape it.

Equivalence

A similar technique is the 'equivalence technique' whereby respondents are asked to identify their point of indifference between keeping alive a group of people in a state of fairly good health and a larger group, whose size is determined by the respondent, of less well people.

Time trade-off

With this method, the technique is to vary the length of time in each health state with treatment choice. For example, the respondent is presented with two alternatives and asked to select the more preferred. Alternative 1 offers the respondent a particular health outcome for a specified length of time followed by death, and alternative 2 offers a different outcome for a different length of time. The time is varied until the respondent is indifferent between the two alternatives.

This technique then requires patients to judge how long a period in one state of health could be 'traded' for a different period in another state of health. The assumption underlying this concept is that the better their state of health, the shorter period of life people would accept as a 'trade-off' for longer survival in a less desirable state.

All utility scales achieve interval scales. Research has found that subjects find the trade-off techniques the easiest of the utility measures, the standard gamble has been found to be more difficult for people, and the rating scale the most difficult. One main criticism of these techniques is that disease sufferers probably assign more positive utilities to states of ill health than normal subjects in hypothetical disease states. Very elderly persons may feel that a frail and painful existence is just as valuable to them as someone else's apparently healthier state.

Such models suffer from several limitations. They have not been adequately tested for validity and reliability, and they rarely ask sufferers themselves to make ratings. Judgements are usually made by 'experts' (e.g. doctors, nurses and medical students). These assume that people are rational when assessing quality of life, and that individual value judgements are not interfering with their ratings. It is also difficult to quantify quality of life, which is a multidimensional concept, in terms of one figure.

3
The measurement of functional ability

There are a number of methodological techniques available for measuring function: direct physical tests of function, direct observation of behaviour and interviews with the person concerned or a third party. Each method has its limitations, as has been indicated. Direct observation is rarely used because it is so time consuming. Direct tests of functioning, such as range-of-limb movement, grip strength, walking time or standards such as joint swelling, pain scores, morning stiffness, erythrocyte sedimentation rate and joint counts, while objective, may not necessarily give an accurate indication of ability or performance. Grip strength will tell you how much a patient can and will squeeze a bag on a particular day. Patients may be more concerned with subjective feelings and reductions in activities associated with daily living.

Most measures of functional disability are self-report methods. Respondents are asked to report limitations on their activities. Sometimes researchers do not wish to use a long scale to measure functional status, usually because their questionnaires are already fairly lengthy, and they therefore prefer single-item questions. One well-known example is the UK government's annual General Household Survey which limits its measure of functional status to questions such as:

Do you have any longstanding illness, disability or infirmity? By long-standing I mean anything that has troubled you over a period of time or that is likely to affect you over a period of time?

(IF YES):

(a) What is the matter with you?
(b) Does this illness or disability limit your activities in any way?
                    (Office of Population Censuses and Surveys 1987)

The main criticism levied at this type of measure is: how limited does a person have to be to answer 'yes'? Subjectivity is involved: people who are short sighted might reply 'yes' or they might not define their condition as a 'longstanding illness, disability or infirmity' or as limiting. Also, people who are used to their conditions and the restrictions they impose may no longer define them as limiting. However, if a measure of perceived health status is required, rather than objective morbidity indicators, then this inherent subjectivity is the strength of the measure.

There are many measures of functional ability. Only those which are either most well tested for validity and reliability, of current topical interest, are frequently used or are potentially applicable in Europe as well as in the USA, are presented in detail. Other scales which are less well tested, but which are popular or are frequently used, are also presented but in less detail (e.g. the Katz Index of Activities of Daily Living, Barthel Index and the Karnofsky Scale).

There are also several available measures of broader health status which incorporate measures of functional ability. These are discussed in chapter 4 along with other broad health-status measures.

Measures of functional ability – e.g. self-care (e.g. eating, bathing, dressing), mobility and physical activities – are frequently used measures because they are socially relevant and interpretable. However, self-care limitations are rare in a general population – less than 0.5 per cent report limitations in eating, dressing, bathing or using the toilet due to poor health. Thus in studies of the general population these items should be selected sparingly in contrast to studies of the severely ill or very elderly where self-care measures may be more appropriate. Broad measures of function are also likely to miss specific effects of disease and generic measures should be supplemented with highly focused measures of disease impact.

Most measures narrowly focus on a range of mobility, domestic and self-care tasks, often, however, ignoring financial, emotional and social needs which may be equally or more important. Measures of physical functioning and activity limitations do not always provide assessments of functioning in everyday social roles, mental functioning, sexual functioning, pain and comfort. More meaningful aspects of household roles are also largely ignored: for example, the effect of the condition on the time taken to perform chores such as cleaning, cooking, shopping, errands, child-care and other caring roles. Assessments of patients' satisfaction and choice with regard to level of functioning are seldom made. People may prefer to have a strip wash rather than to risk slipping while getting into the bath. On scales of function it is generally assumed that respondents achieving a low score due to immobility necessarily have a poorer quality of life than a patient with a higher score. Thus someone who is wheelchair bound might have a low ADL score, despite the fact s/he may be receiving good-quality social support.

Moreover, most scales have been developed on the basis of professionals' (e.g. doctors') judgements about essential abilities for daily living. Berg *et al.* (1976) asked 150 health workers to assign weight from 0 to 10 for 50 listed abilities or functions; open-ended questions to elicit functions not listed were also used. Serious problems were documented in finding simple and meaningful terms to describe functional loss to many respondents. Respondents assigned the largest average values to ability to use one's mental abilities, to see, to think clearly, to love and be loved, to make decisions for oneself, to live at home, to walk, to maintain contact with family and friends, and to talk. Although the sample was limited to health workers, the results indicate a need to consider lay person's judgements of essential functions and to include these in measures of health outcomes.

The problem of measuring functional disability is compounded by conceptual difficulties and interactive factors. One of the major problems with using a functional index is that different patients may react differently to apparently similar levels of physical impairment, depending on their expectations, priorities, goals, social-support networks and so on. Functional disability, like dependency, is a multi-dimensional concept which may relate to physical, mental, cognitive, social, economic or environmental factors (Wilkin 1987). Thus it is an interactive concept – it is not a necessary consequence of impairment but perhaps, for example, of the siting of bathrooms, toilets and other facilities and the necessity for negotiating stairs. In terms of dependency, severity might be a function of the existence of aids or the frequency and timing of help. Perceptions of severity with both disability and dependency will also be influenced by previous history and expectations for the future. Meaning apart, most scales are not sensitive enough as they simply ask respondents whether they have no or some difficulty with a task, or whether they are unable to perform it at all. The problem emerges of how limited does one have to be to answer in the affirmative? More sensitive scales with greater response choices based on degrees of severity require development.

Also there are often differing viewpoints of how people ought to be performing, for instance, on the part of surgeon and patients. The patient may want to walk without aids or limp, whilst the surgeon may regard 'walking with aids and limp' as indicative of a satisfactory outcome.

Finally, caution is needed when deciding on which measures to use. Measures tend to be developed, administered and validated on one of two types of samples – people living in the community or in institutions. The measures are not necessarily interchangeable between samples. The measures must be appropriate for the population type. Many measures have been developed to be optimally suitable for a particular age group and may be inappropriate for use with other age groups.

The Older American's Resources and Services Schedule (OARS): Multi-dimensional Functional Assessment Questionnaire

The OARS Multidimensional Functional Assessment Questionnaire was developed in order to measure the level of functioning and need for services of older people. It was developed at Duke University Center for the Study of Ageing and Human Development (Fillenbaum 1978; Fillenbaum and Smyer 1981). The measure was developed for use with adults aged 55 and over and should be restricted to this age group. Gatz et al. (1987) tested OARS on a sample of over 1000 people aged 26–86 and reported that the global test scores can be misleading when applied to different age groups. It can be used with community or institutional samples. When used with institutionalized samples some questions are omitted, and institution-relevant items are added.

OARS measures five dimensions of personal functioning, including mental impairment. Despite its popularity, little work has been done on the measurement properties of the mental-health scale.

The numerous applications of the OARS during its construction are described in the OARS handbook (Fillenbaum 1978). One of the most well-known studies using the OARS questionnaire was the survey of social support in relation to mortality carried out in Durham, North Carolina (Blazer 1982). This was based on 331 people aged 65 years and over, taken from a wider community sample survey of 997 people. This sub-sample was followed up 30 months after baseline interview which assessed functional status, social support, depressive symptoms, physical-health status and cognitive functioning, stressful life events and cigarette smoking. Increased mortality risk was found for those with impaired social support and social interaction. The OARS questionnaire has been widely used throughout the USA and has also been used in Australia. Two Spanish translations are available for use with Spanish-speaking people in America.

Administration time is on average 45 minutes but probably takes an hour generally to administer. The main limitation of OARS is its length. A shorter version of OARS is available, known as the Functional Assessment Inventory (FAI), although this still takes approximately 35 minutes to administer. The FAI contains the functional assessment items, but not the detailed service-use items. Interviewer training, which takes two days, is recommended. Its administration is also explained in a manual which can be purchased from the authors.

Content

The questionnaire consists of two independent sections. Part A assesses functional status in relation to social, economic, mental and physical health, and activities of daily living. Interviewers also make ratings of ability. The responses to the items in each area are summarized on a six-point scale (e.g. level of functioning: 1 = excellent to 6 = totally impaired). These five ratings yield a profile showing concomitant functioning across the five areas. Part B is a services assessment that directs enquiry into 24 generically defined services, determining for each the current use, the extent of use in the past six months, the type of service provider and perceived need. There is also a demographic section. Information is sought from the respondent, proxy interviews are permitted. If sub-questions are included, the total number of items asked is 120. Examples of the items are:

Can you get to places out of walking distance?

2 Without help (can travel alone on buses, taxis, or drive your own car).
1 With some help (need someone to help you or go with you when travelling).
0 Or are you unable to travel unless emergency arrangements are made for a specialized vehicle like an ambulance?
– Not answered.

Can you go shopping for groceries or clothes (assuming subject has transportation)?

2 Without help (taking care of all shopping needs yourself, assuming you had transportation).
1 With some help (need someone to go with you on all shopping trips).
0 Or are you completely unable to go shopping?
– Not answered.

Can you prepare your own meals?

2 Without help (plan and cook full meals yourself).
1 With some help (can prepare some things but unable to cook full meals yourself).
0 Or are you completely unable to prepare any meals?
– Not answered.

Can you do your own housework?

2 Without help (can scrub floors, etc.).
1 With some help (can do light housework but need help with heavy work).
0 Or are you completely unable to do any housework?
– Not answered.

Scoring

There are various methods of aggregation. The 1–6 ratings on each of the five scales may be summed (5: excellent functioning in each area to 30: total overall impairment), although summing is problematic as was indicated earlier. Alternatively, the number of areas of functioning that are impaired can be counted. To do this, it is necessary first to establish which level of functioning indicates impairment. Ratings of 1 and 2 may be combined and compared with ratings of 3–6 (i.e. non-impaired versus impaired) or the contrast may be between ratings of 1–3 and 4–6. Summed over areas, this yields a 6-class system (0 areas of functioning impaired to 5 areas impaired). A more complex classification based on a trichotomized scale (1+2/3+4/5+6) which takes account of both number of areas of impairment and severity of impairment has also been developed; full details are contained in the handbook. It is also possible to examine the responses to each individual question and treat the items as separate units. For clinical purposes it might be important to maintain the distinctions but not for population purposes.

However, a classification based on summed information assumes that areas are equivalent; at present the validity of this assumption has not been established. Consequently a classification system that maintains distinctions between areas may be preferred.

Validity

OARS and the shorter FAI were extensively tested for validity at the various stages of its development (Fillenbaum 1978; Cairl et al. 1983). Both instruments appear to have face and content validity, although discriminant and predictive validity have not yet been adequately tested.

Criterion validity was tested on 33 patients from a family medical practice. Spearman correlation between separate criterion ratings and the economic items was 0.68, 0.67 for mental health, 0.82 for physical health, and 0.89 for self-care ability. On another study of 82 community residents, the Spearmen correlation between independent psychiatrists' ratings and the mental-health items was 0.62, and between physicians' assistants ratings and the physical-health items was 0.70. Detailed results for reliability and validity of OARS can be found in Fillenbaum (1978) and Fillenbaum and Smyer (1981), and results for the FAI can be found in Cairl et al. (1983).

Reliability

OARS and the FAI has been extensively tested for reliability. Tests of agreement of the raters' assessments have been carried out involving eleven raters who assessed 30 patients. Intraclass correlations ranged from 0.66 for physical health to 0.87 for self-care. Raters were in complete agreement for 74 per cent of the ratings (Fillenbaum 1978). Reliability ratings of the Community Service Questionnaire gave inter-rater Kendall coefficients of concordance between 0.70 and 0.93. Test-retest reliability, conducted 12–18 months apart, gave correlations of between 0.47 and 1.00. Five-week test-retest correlations based on ratings of 30 elderly people gave results of 0.82 for the physical Activities of Daily Living (ADL) questions, such as personal care, 0.71 for the Instrumental Activities of Daily Living (IADL) questions, such as housework, and 0.79 for the economic resources items. For social resources the correlation was 0.71 and for subjective questions it was 0.53. Coefficients for life satisfaction and mental health were lower: 0.42 and 0.32 respectively.

Although much of the data on reliability and validity refers to previous versions of the instrument, the OARS appears to be a superior measure to most others. It was unhesitatingly recommended by McDowell and Newell (1987) in their review of measures. On the other hand it has been criticized for the excessive number of sub-items and the lengthy period of administration (Perlman 1987).

The Stanford Arthritis Center Health Assessment Questionnaire (HAQ)

Fries *et al.* (1980) developed the HAQ on the basis that outcome should be measured in terms of the patient's value system. Functional ability (e.g. the ability to walk) is a component of this but sedimentation rate is not. The framework used for the development of the HAQ was based on the belief that a patient desires to be alive, free of pain, functioning normally, experiencing minimal treatment toxicity, and financially solvent. Patient outcome was thus represented by (1) death, (2) discomfort, (3) disability, (4) therapeutic toxicity, (5) dollar cost.

In the process of developing this measure 62 potential questions were selected from questionnaires in use in the rheumatic-diseases field and elsewhere, including the Uniform Database for Rheumatic Diseases (Fries *et al.* 1974; Convery *et al.* 1977); the Barthel Index (Mahoney and Barthel 1965); the ADL (Katz *et al.* 1963). Testing the measure for reliability and validity with patients with rheumatoid arthritis reduced the measure to 21 questions, grouped into nine components, and graded in ordinal fashion from 0 to 3. Individual items with correlations of 0.85 or higher were eliminated in the interests of conciseness, on the assumption that this suggested redundancy between components. Correlations of remaining items range between 0.35 and 0.65 (Fries *et al.* 1980). The resulting instrument was subsequently administered in more than two dozen settings.

The HAQ is suitable for use in community settings and has been administered to patients with rheumatoid and osteoarthritis, systemic lupus and ankylosing spondylitis.

It is relatively coherent and concise and is self-administered so does not rely on skilled personnel to administer (it is therefore relatively cheap). Administration takes 5–8 minutes and manual scoring can be completed within a minute.

Content

Functional ability is measured by nine components: dressing and grooming, rising, eating, walking, hygiene, reach, grip, outside activity and sexual activity. Each of these components consists of one or more relevant questions. Pain, discomfort, drug toxicity and financial costs are also assessed. Examples of questions are:

Are you able to:
Dress yourself, including tying shoelaces and doing buttons?
Stand up from an armless chair?
Get in and out of bed?
Walk outdoors on flat ground?
Do chores such as vacuuming, housework or light gardening?

The range of answers is, 'without any difficulty; with some difficulty; with much difficulty; unable to do'.

Scoring

In relation to functional ability, the ordinal scoring of 0–3 is based on the following scale: without difficulty = 0, with some difficulty = 1, with much difficulty = 2 and unable to do = 3. The index is calculated by the addition of scores and then dividing the score by the total number of components answered. The authors reported reluctance among patients to report sexual activity (Fries et al. 1980), and thus some investigators omit this item (Fitzpatrick et al. 1988).

The scales of pain, discomfort and drug toxicity ranges from 0 to 3. Questions concerning the severity of pain range from none = 0 to severe = 3. The scale for discomfort comprises better = 1, the same = 2 or worse = 3. The drug toxicity index is composed of questions about the adverse effects from drugs and treatment ranging from none = 0 to severe = 3. Initial tests for validity and reliability revealed weak results, and this component requires further testing (Fries et al. 1980).

In the personal-cost section (applicable to private health care systems), medical and surgical costs are calculated for the past year. The number and type of medications, X-rays, surgery, physician and paramedical visits, appliances, number of laboratory tests, and hospitalizations are detailed. The average cost in the area covered by the research team (Stanford, California) was determined and used for the computation of the dollar values. This section can be applied only in countries and areas where costs are known. Social costs are calculated by determining changes in employment, income, the need to employ domestic help, the cost of transport for medical care and all arthritis-related costs over the past twelve months (Fries *et al.* 1980). The cost questions have not yet been satisfactorily tested; initial tests for validity suffered from poor patient recall.

Fitzpatrick *et al.* (1989), in their comparison of the HAQ and the Functional Limitation Profile (FLP) (derived from the Sickness Impact Profile), reported that nothing appeared to be achieved in relation to precision by the complex scoring system utilized by the FLP in comparison with the simpler ordinal assumptions of the HAQ.

Validity

It has been extensively validated. Correlations of the HAQ against observed patient performance ranged from fair to high (0.47–0.88) (Fries *et al.* 1980; Fries *et al.* 1982; Fries 1983; Kirwan and Reeback 1983).

Several studies have tested the validity of the HAQ, in particular by correlation of the results of the HAQ with the Arthritis Impact Measurement Scale (AIMS) (Fries *et al.* 1982; Brown *et al.* 1984). These two measures were shown to measure the same dimensions of disability; the correlation coefficient reported by Fries *et al.* (1982) was 0.91. Inter-correlations between the three parts of each instrument relating to physical disability, psychological state and pain were high and those across these three dimensions were weak. Patient self-assessed global arthritis scores were also strongly associated with disability score and less strongly to pain. These correlations are consistent with current knowledge within the speciality of rheumatology, that disability is a large component of arthritic patients' concerns.

A recent study in the UK by Fitzpatrick *et al.* (1988) of 105 patients with rheumatoid arthritis reported high inter-measure correlations between the HAQ, the Functional Limitation Profile (FLP) (Charlton *et al.* 1983), and between observations of grip strength and the articular index (e.g. the correlations between grip strength and the HAQ on two occasions were –0.73 and –0.68). The HAQ appears to be a valid measure of function in rheumatoid arthritis.

Principal components analysis has shown factor loadings along the first 'disability' component, which explains 65 per cent of the variance, and a second component with positive loadings for fine activities of the upper extremity and negative loadings for weight bearing actions of the lower extremity, which explains an additional 10 per cent of the variance (Fries *et al.* 1980; 1982). From this, it was inferred that the resulting disability index (an equal weight sum) is well focused and appropriate for measuring overall arthritis severity.

The HAQ was reported in early studies to be sensitive to change (Fries 1983). Fitzpatrick *et al.* (1989), in their UK study, reported that the HAQ performed better than the FLP in relation to specificity and sensitivity (detection of change over time), although at best this can only be said to be moderate. The large standard deviations in the scores of both measures indicated the presence of many 'false positives' for both improvement and deterioration. Further testing is required for its sensitivity.

Reliability

The earliest tests for reliability were reported by Fries *et al.* (1980). In addition to the reporting of mean values, these included correlations of HAQ scores with the results of direct observations by a nurse of patients' performance of 15 household and personal-care tasks, mobility and grip; and of self-administered and interview-based HAQ completion. These early tests were based on just 20 patient volunteers attending a rheumatoid-arthritis clinic. The correlations for individual items for self-administration versus interview-administered HAQ range from average (or 'respectable') at 0.56 to excellent 0.85. The corresponding correlations for the disability score was 0.85, indicating good reliability for this component.

The inter-method correlations ranged from average at 0.47 to excellent at 0.88. The weaker items (e.g. reach) were subsequently reworded to minimize variability in responses – e.g. this question originally read 'reach and get down heavy objects'. People's ideas of 'heavy' varied, so respondents are now asked about a standardized item: 'reach and get down a 5lb. bag of sugar which is above your head'. The authors also compared overall questionnaire and evaluator agreement; these agreed exactly on 59 per cent of the responses and were within one point in 93 per cent of cases (the weighted Kappa statistic result, using rank disagreement rates, was 0.52, implying 'moderate' agreement).

Fries *et al.* (1982) reported mean values from a diverse English-speaking community population of 331 respondents suffering from rheumatoid arthritis. The authors also reported the test-retest correlation of 0.98, based on this population. The mean values showed stability on repeat testing. Responses are similar when the instrument is self-completed, administered by a nurse or doctor.

The HAQ is a good measure of function and has been extensively tested for reliability and validity. It is concise, sensitive to change, can be self- or interviewer-administered and is suitable for use in the community. However, it is really only suitable for use with chronically ill patients and the questions relate to negative health. It has been extensively used among clinicians in the USA and UK.

The Arthritis Impact Measurement Scale (AIMS)

The AIMS Scale was developed by Meenan *et al.* (1980), partly adapted from Katz's Index of Daily Living, the Rand Health Insurance Study Scales and The Quality of Well-Being Scale (Patrick *et al.* 1973a; Brook *et al.* 1979a, 1979b; Ware *et al.* 1979; Bush 1984). This measure aims to assess patient outcome in arthritis and other chronic diseases. It covers physical, social and emotional well-being. The advantages of AIMS are that it is well tested for reliability and validity; it is concise and can be self-administered or interview based; it is sensitive to change and it is suitable for use in the community. As with the HAQ, the disadvantages of AIMS are that it is really only suitable for use with chronically ill patients and the questions relate to negative health. AIMS is extensively used in USA, but less in UK and Europe. It is self-administered and takes approximately 15 minutes to complete.

Content

AIMS assesses nine dimensions of health and functional ability: mobility, physical activity (walking, bending, lifting), activities of daily living, dexterity, household activities (management of money, medication, housekeeping), pain, social activity, depression and anxiety. An additional 19 items cover general health, health perceptions and demographic details (e.g. a visual analogue item that assesses the respondent's overall health rating; perceived susceptibility to illness; other diseases present and treatment). Typical questions from the AIMS are:

Do you have to stay indoors most or all of the day because of your health   Yes/No

Do you have trouble bending, lifting or stooping because of your health?   Yes/No

Can you easily turn a key in a lock?   Yes/No

How much help do you need in getting dressed?   No help at all/only need help in tying shoes/need help in getting dressed

During the past month, how much of the time have you enjoyed the things you do?   All of the time/most of the time/a good bit of the time/some of the time/a little of the time/none of the time?

During the past month, how much of the time have you felt tense or 'high strung?'   All of the time/most of the time/a good bit of the time/some of the time/a little of the time/none of the time?

Some items require just yes/no answers and others are scaled.

Scoring

To achieve the item scores some recording is required as the questionnaire items are worded and coded to avoid response bias. The AIMS instrument is composed of 45 items; these are summed into nine scales. A 'normalization procedure' converts scores into the range of 0–10, with 0 representing good 'health status' and 10 representing poor 'health status'.

For each scale, the items are listed in Guttman order so that a respondent indicating disability on one item will also indicate disability on section items falling below it. In scoring AIMS Guttman characteristics are ignored and each item is scored separately, with higher scores indicating greater limitation. Most questions refer to problems experienced within the last month. No item weights are used. A total health-status score can be derived by adding the values for the six scales: mobility, physical activity, household activity, dexterity, pain and depression. The scale is ordinal in type. It has been described as superior to other applications of Guttman scaling (McDowell and Newell 1987).

Validity

The AIMS is a good measure of function and has been extensively tested for reliability and validity (Meenan et al. 1980; Meenan et al. 1982, 1984; Meenan 1982; 1985; Brown et al. 1984). All nine AIMS scales have been reported to be highly correlated with physician-produced estimates of health status, and specific scales correlated highly with standard measures of physical function. The content of AIMS overlaps with the Health Assessment Questionnaire (HAQ) by about 65 per cent. In all cases, however, the actual questionnaire items are different. Both instruments contain a single horizontal visual analogue scale assessing the patient's perception of arthritis status, providing a 'global health estimate'. A study administering both instruments (HAQ and AIMS) to patients with rheumatoid arthritis demonstrated that the different scales measure similar dimensions of health status in this type of chronic disease. The instruments were highly correlated, providing convergent validation for the existence of three relatively discrete components of health status: pain, physical disability and psychological status (Brown et al. 1984).

All nine scales were weakly to moderately (all significant) correlated with two physician-derived general standards of health status (American

Rheumatism Association Function: r between 0.24 and 0.52 and disease status: r between 0.14 and 0.52). AIMS scales were also correlated with clinical rheumatology standards: walking time, grip strength, joint count, range of motion. The items measuring physical well-being (mobility, physical activity, dexterity, household activities, activities of daily living) were more highly correlated with these physical standards than were the AIMS psychological and social scales (e.g. dexterity correlated highly with grip strength; mobility and physical activity were most strongly related to walking time).

The second part of the validity testing involved a series of factor analyses designed to determine whether the items in the AIMS scales would group together in a consistent and coherent way. The single-scale factor analyses demonstrated that each set of AIMS items except household activities loaded strongly on a single factor. This indicated that the group items represented a coherent scale. The nine AIMS items were grouped into three discrete factors in relation to health status: physical function, psychological function and pain.

More recent developments by its authors include a four-factor and a five-factor model, developed from studies of 360 rheumatoid arthritis patients, on the grounds that these are more likely to reflect the major dimensions of health status and represent a fuller assessment of health status. In the five-factor model, the physical dimension of AIMS exhibits separate upper-extremity and lower-extremity components. The fourth factor, primarily represented by the pain scale, reflects the added arthritis symptom measure (Mason et al. 1988). The five-component model also facilitates statistical analysis, such as multiple regression, in which five distinct components are preferable to the original nine more highly inter-correlated scales for use as explanatory variables. Each AIMS scale can also continue to be used alone. More work still remains to be done to develop and test the five-component model.

The sensitivity of AIMS was assessed by comparing it with standard clinical outcome measures (joint counts for tenderness and swelling, grip strength, physician assessments of disease activity and functional class) in a double-blind, multi-centre clinical drug trial based on 161 patients (Meenan et al. 1984). Using AIMS, differences between treatments were found for physical activity, anxiety, depression, pain and the overall impact using the visual analogue scale item. The findings were consistent with other studies of the same treatments and demonstrated that AIMS is sensitive enough to detect clinically meaningful differences in treatment outcomes. It was as sensitive as traditional clinical measures and also indicated additional differences not detected by standard approaches.

AIMS has been adapted and used to measure and compare health status across chronic disease groups (rheumatoid arthritis, cardiac disease, diabetes, hypertension, breast cancer, chronic obstructive pulmonary disease). Statistically significant differences emerged across all disease groups with the exception of activities of daily living, anxiety and depression. Thus AIMS may be applied to a range of conditions (Brown et al. 1984; Meenan 1985).

Since its initial development the three-component model AIMS has been used in many studies (Kazis et al. 1983; Meenan et al. 1984; Kazis et al. 1988; Mason et al. 1988). Its applications have been predominantly in clinical settings (with arthritis and rheumatism patients) as an assessment of outcome after therapy.

Reliability

AIMS was tested on a sample of 625 English-speaking patients with various rheumatic diseases, drawn from 15 different clinical establishments in 10 US states. No major problems emerged with comprehension or administration.

Coefficients of scalability and reliability on all nine AIMS scales exceeded 0.60 and 0.90 respectively for all but the household-activity scale. The test-retest correlation across all nine scale items was 0.87. These results indicated good internal consistency, strong hierarchical scale properties and test-retest stability.

The tests for reliability and validity were repeated on a variety of subjects in different demographic, functional and diagnostic categories. Most reliability coefficients were reported as meeting or exceeding accepted criteria. The pattern of validity correlations were maintained (Meenan et al. 1980; 1982; Meenan 1982; Brown et al. 1984).

In sum, AIMS has good measurement properties, has been extensively tested for validity, and the identified dimensions explain the majority of illness impact estimated by patients. However, the specificity of this instrument makes it unsuitable for use with groups other than the chronically ill and is recommended as an outcome indicator for use with arthritis patients.

The Index of Activities of Daily Living (ADL)

One of the best known and oldest of the disability scales is the Activities of Daily Living (ADL) index developed by Katz et al. (1963; 1966; 1968; 1970; 1973; 1976). They designed the Index of Activities of Daily Living in order to describe, for clinical purposes, the states of elderly patients.

Content

The index consists of a rating form that is completed by a therapist or other observer. In each of the activities assessed the patient is rated by the observer on a three-point scale of independence for each activity. Examples from the evaluation form are:

Bathing
Receives no assistance (gets in and out of tub by self if tub is usual means of bathing) _____
Receives assistance in bathing only one part of the body (such as back of a leg) _____
Receives assistance in bathing more than one part of the body (or not bathed) _____

Dressing
Gets clothes and gets completely dressed without assistance _____
Gets clothes and gets dressed without assistance except for assistance in tying shoes _____
Receives assistance in getting clothes or in getting dressed, or stays partly or completely undressed _____

Continence
Controls urination and bowel movement completely by self _____
Has occasional accidents _____
Supervision helps keep urine or bowel control; catheter is used, or is incontinent _____

Feeding
Feeds self without assistance _____
Feeds self except for getting assistance in cutting meat or buttering bread _____
Receives assistance in feeding or is fed partly or completely by using tubes or intravenous fluids _____

The authors later developed a survey instrument for obtaining health-status data containing questions about the need for and use of health services and attitudes towards medical care. Five categories of 'need' were defined and ranked: no disability, restricted activity with no chronic conditions, restricted activity with chronic condition, mobility limitations and bed disability. These were chosen to permit comparisons with existing national surveys (Katz *et al.* 1973).

Scoring

Patients are graded on ordinal scales by interviewers in relation to their ability in bathing, dressing, transferring (e.g. to chair), toileting, continence and feeding. Scores on individual scales were summed, all items being treated as equally important, thus yielding a single total score. On the basis of more than 2,000 evaluations of states of patients, the authors observed that these functions decreased in order. They claimed to have a measure of fundamental biological functions, a claim questioned by those using Guttman scales (Williams *et al.* 1976).

The first stage in the scoring involves translating the three-point scales into a dependent/independent classification. The patients' overall performance is then summarized on an eight-point scale:

A Independent in feeding, continence, transferring, going to toilet, dressing and bathing
B Independent in all but one of these functions
C Independent in all but bathing and one additional function
D Independent in all but bathing, dressing and one additional function
E Independent in all but bathing, dressing, going to toilet and one additional function
F Independent in all but bathing, dressing, going to toilet, transferring and one additional function
G Dependent in all six functions
Other   Dependent in at least two functions, but not classifiable as C, D, E or F.

Full definitions of activities are given by Katz *et al.* (1970).

The use of a single index means loss of information about variability, because difference patterns of restriction, with different implications, can be reduced to the same score.

Validity

Despite the scale's widespread popularity among clinicians worldwide, there is little evidence of the validity of the scale. Katz *et al.* (1970) administered the ADL and other instruments to 270 chronically ill patients. The ADL correlated weakly to moderately with a mobility scale (0.50) and with a house-confinement scale (0.39).

The index of ADL was shown to predict the long-term course and social adaptation of patients with a number of conditions, including strokes and hip fractures, and was used to evaluate out-patient treatment for rheumatoid arthritis (Katz *et al.* 1964; 1966; 1968). It has also been shown to predict mortality (Brorsson and Asberg 1984). There is other evidence of its predictive validity, reported by Katz and Akpom (1976). However, such concise indices tend to be insensitive to small changes in disease severity and to focus on physical-performance measures. It is also of limited value in community surveys of elderly people because, like other short scales, it does not take adaptation to environment into account. It apparently underestimates dysfunction in community populations (Spector *et al.* 1987).

Reliability

Little testing for reliability has been carried out; this is again surprising given the popularity of this scale, particularly by clinicians. Katz *et al.* (1963) assessed inter-rater reliability; they reported that discrepancies between raters occurred in one in twenty observations.

A Swedish study of Guttman analyses on 100 patients yielded coefficients of scalability of 0.74–0.88, suggesting that the index is a successful cumulative scale (Brorsson and Asberg 1984). More evidence of the ADL's reliability and validity is required.

The Katz is one of the earliest indices for use in evaluating care of elderly and chronically ill patients. It is a popular and useful index with a restricted range of patients. However, the range of disabilities included in the instrument is not comprehensive and thus the populations to which it can be administered are restricted. The single index also means that the information derived from the index is limited.

Townsend's Disability Scale

Townsend's Disability Scale is a concise index which is frequently used in community surveys of the elderly in the UK. It comprises a list of activities of daily living, derived from early research on the disabled of all ages in the UK and USA (Haber 1968; Sainsbury 1973) and Townsend's own early survey work on the elderly (Townsend 1962; Shanas *et al.* 1968). It was also used in Townsend's later poverty survey (Townsend 1979). However, little work has been carried out on its reliability and validity apart from initial piloting based on these early studies. Moreover, this early work was not very thorough. Sainsbury (1973) states that the list of tasks of daily living initially selected were chosen on the basis of a 'subjective' decision 'of the more important daily and social activities'. Its advantages are its brevity and acceptability to elderly people.

Content

The index deliberately focuses on a narrow range of activities, in order that the concepts underlying them are generally applicable to a wide section of the population and for ease of application within a survey framework of the general population:

(a) activities which maintain personal existence, such as drinking, eating, evacuating, exercising, sleeping, hearing, washing and dressing

(b) activities which provide the means to fulfil these personal acts, such as obtaining food, preparing meals, providing and cleaning a home.

The scale asks respondents if they have difficulty doing the following tasks, (none = 0, some difficulty = 1 or unable to do alone = 2) washing all over, cutting own toenails, running to catch a bus, carrying heavy shopping, going up/down stairs, doing heavy housework, preparing a hot meal, reaching a jug from an overhead shelf and tying a good knot in a piece of string. It can be self- or interviewer-administered, is easily completed and concise. For example:

Do you or would you have any difficulty (or find it troublesome, exhausting or worrying)

(a) **Washing down (whether in bath or not)?**
(b) **Removing a jug, say, from an overhead shelf?**
(c) **Tying a good knot in string?**
(d) **Cutting toenails?**

The remaining questions are not asked of children under the age of 10 or the bedfast:

(e) **Running to catch a bus?**
(f) **Going up/down stairs?**
(g) **Going shopping and carrying a full basket of shopping in each hand?**
(h) **Doing heavy housework?**
(i) **Preparing a hot meal?**

Scoring

Difficulty with each activity is given equal weighting; changes in individual capacity from day to day and season to season are ignored. 'No difficulty' is scored as zero, 'with some difficulty' is scored as 1, and the score is 2 if the reply was 'unable to do alone'. The overall score has a range of 0–18. Townsend, as a result of early validation work, regards people with a score of zero as having no disability, 1–2 as slightly affected, 3–6 some disability, 7–10 as appreciable disability and 11–18 as severe/very severe. The basis for this does not appear to have been tested any further. It is a limited index, covering a narrow range of activities.

Validity and reliability

Neither of the studies from which the scale is derived provides details of the initial testing of the measure (Haber 1968; Sainsbury 1973).

There are numerous examples in the UK of applications of the scale, particularly by Vetter *et al.* (e.g. Vetter *et al.* 1982; Vetter and Ford 1989).

The scale is popular, although further and extensive testing for reliability and validity is still required.

Adaptations

There are numerous adaptations of the scale. Some of the items are not appropriate for use with a frail population, e.g. 'running to catch a bus'. The limitations of this scale have led to adaptation of the scale by many researchers, in terms of adding other activities of daily living and increasing the range of responses: no difficulty with the task, slight, moderate or severe difficulty, unable to do alone, and unable to do at all (even with help) (Bowling *et al.* 1988). The scale was extended by the latter authors to include all the following tasks:

Getting in/out of bed
Transferring from a chair/wheelchair
Going up/down stairs
Getting on/off toilet
Getting in/out of bath
Getting about in-doors
Getting about out-doors
Using public transport

Washing self/shaving (men)
Bathing self
Dressing self
Brush/comb hair
Wash hair
Cutting toe-nails

Cooking/prepare meal
Housework
Laundry
Shopping
Doing odd jobs

Two other items were initially included, brushing or managing teeth and handling money, but these appeared ambiguous. They were excluded after factor analysis. On the basis of community surveys with 662 people aged 85 and over living in London, and almost 700 people aged 65-plus living in Essex and London, inter-item correlations coefficients between tasks ranged from around 0.13 (this was for shopping and managing teeth or dentures which would not be expected necessarily to correlate highly) to around 0.74 (for difficulties with washing self and with dressing self which would be expected to correlate more highly); split half reliability: 0.78–

0.91 between samples. The inter-item correlation (alpha) for the personal-care-task section was 0.70–0.75; for the domestic–task section was 0.80–0.85; and for the mobility section was 0.81–0.89. Tests for validity, with the Health Assessment Questionnaire as a gold standard, are ongoing.

A similar scale has also been developed by the Institute for Economic and Social Research at York University and used in a wide range of surveys (Morton-Williams 1979). Their scale encompasses a wider range of self-care activities than the original Townsend scale, with rankings of: able to do easily, with a little difficulty, with a lot of difficulty, unable to do without someone helping, unable to do even with someone helping (the latter ranking is not always included). However, testing on this scale is also incomplete.

Another adaptation of the scale has been undertaken by Bond and Carstairs (1982) in their survey of 5,000 elderly people in Scotland. These authors distinguished between functional criteria for dependency (mobility, self-care and home-care capacity) and clinical criteria for dependency (incontinence, mental state), and they attempted to measure these. They selected items from the original Sainsbury scale, on the basis of inter-item correlations, which were then subjected to a Guttman scaling analysis. The items selected were based on a hierarchical concept: having difficulty with an activity is associated with having difficulty with earlier scale items. The items classified as mobility incapacity were difficulty/ability travelling by bus, walking outside, getting up from chair (coefficient of reproducibility: 0.97); self-care incapacity included difficulty/ability washing hair, self, bathing; dressing, put on shoes and socks/stockings (coefficient of reproducibility: 0.99); and home-care incapacity included: difficulty/ability: doing heavy shopping; washing clothes; preparing and cooking meals; ironing clothes; light housework; making bed (coefficient of reproducibility: 0.96).

The Karnofsky Performance Scale

The Karnofsky Performance Scale emphasizes physical performance and dependency. It was originally designed for use with lung cancer patients in relation to assessing palliative treatments (Karnofsky et al. 1948). It is a simple scale from 1 to 100 (normal–moribund). It was developed for use in clinical settings. The scale is heavily weighted towards the physical dimensions of quality of life, rather than social and psychological dimensions. Patients are assigned to categories by a clinician or other health-care professional. It is widely used in the USA and Europe.

A literature review, examining the frequency of measurement of quality of life in clinical trials of outcome of care in six international cancer journals, showed that only 6 per cent attempted to measure it, and that the vast majority of this 6 per cent used the original performance criteria of Karnofsky (Bardelli and Saracci 1978).

Content

Examples of some of the classifications, which are made by professionals, and scores, are:

Normal; no complaint; no evidence of disease (index: 100).
Requires occasional assistance from others but able to care for most needs (index: 60).
Disabled; requires special care and assistance (index: 40).
Moribund; fatal processes progressing rapidly (index: 10).
Dead; (index: 0).

Scoring

Each component of the scale is given a notional percentage score (100 = normal; 0 = dead). Scores are summed to produce an overall score. The scoring procedure has not been assessed for validity. Various categorizations exist.

There are problems with this method, particularly with the assumption that a patient with a low score due to immobility necessarily has a poorer quality of life than a patient with a higher score, and vice versa. For example, the patient with a poor score may have better social support than a patient with a good score and thus, despite the immobility, may have a better quality of life. Moreover, the Karnofsky ratings are often reported as a mean score, yet there is no evidence that the intervals between the ten categories represent the same degree of dysfunction (O'Brien 1988).

Validity

The disadvantage of the Karnofsky Performance Scale, apart from its crude and therefore limited content, is that it involves categorization of patients by another person. This is a fundamental flaw, given the evidence of discrepancies between patients' and physicians' ratings of functioning and quality of life. In Evans et al.'s (1984) study, for example, there were wide discrepancies between patients' self-assessments, based on the Sickness Impact Profile, and physicians' assessments, based on the Karnofsky index, with the latter rating patients as being less impaired than the former.

Mor et al. (1984) used the scale in a national hospice-evaluation study. They reported that the construct validity of the scale was achieved: it was strongly related to two other independent measures of patient functioning

(Katz's ADL scale and another quality-of-life assessment). It was also able to predict longevity (0.30) in the population of terminally ill cancer patients, thus indicating that it has predictive validity. The Karnofsky Scale is a crude, although successful, predictor of survival. Mor (1987), again in a study of cancer patients (total: 2,046), reported a moderate correlation between the Karnofsky Scale and the Spitzer Quality of Life Index; the correlation was probably moderate because the latter is multidimensional. One of its recent well-known applications has been in the US National Heart Transplantation Study (Evans et al. 1984). Results from this study showed a marked shift in the distribution of Karnofsky scores before and after transplantation. However, it does not measure broader quality of life such as social or emotional well-being and is thus limited as a measure of quality of life.

Reliability

Mor et al. (1984), on the basis of a national hospice evaluation, reported that the inter-rater reliability coefficient of the 47 interviewers employed at test-retests at four-month intervals was 0.97.

Slevin et al. (1988) reported a study involving 108 cancer patients in which two different groups of patients filled in the same collection of instruments, including the Karnofsky index, on a single day, and then daily for five consecutive days. Although the Karnofsky scale was more robust than the other measures tested (Spitzer's Quality of Life Index, the Hospital Anxiety and Depression scale and LASA visual analogue scales), the same score was achieved on only 54 per cent of occasions, despite the fact that only the five top points on the Karnofsky scale were covered.

The reliability and validity of the index have only recently begun to be examined (Hutchinson et al. 1979). The scale's 'numeric' status has not been seriously challenged, and it has generally been uncritically accepted and applied in a large number of clinical settings (Schag et al. 1984). It has even been used in settings where its applicability must be questioned (bone-marrow transplantation in children) (Hinterberger et al. 1987).

The Barthel Index

The Barthel Index was developed by Mahoney and Barthel (1965). It is based on observed functions. The index was developed to measure functional ability before and after intervention treatment, and to indicate the amount of nursing care required. It was designed for use with long-term hospital patients with neuromuscular or musculo-skeletal disorders. It has been used more generally to evaluate treatment outcomes since. The Barthel Index is based on a rating scale completed by a therapist or other observer. The scale takes approximately 30 seconds to score.

Content

The scale covers the following dimensions:

Feeding
Mobility from bed to chair
Personal toilet (washing, etc.)
Getting on/off the toilet
Bathing
Walking on level surface
Going up/down stairs
Dressing
Incontinence (bladder and bowel)

A score of zero is given where the patients cannot meet the defined criterion. It omits tasks of daily living such as cooking and shopping and other everyday tasks essential for life in the community. It thus appears suitable only for institutionalized populations (for whom it was designed).

Granger et al. (1979; 1984) and Fortinsky et al. (1981) have developed extensions of the Barthel Index, covering 15 topics, although insufficient evidence of the reliability and validity of these extensions exists.

Scoring

Different values are assigned to different activities. Individuals are scored on ten activities which are summed to give a score of 0 (totally dependent) to 100 (fully independent). The authors of the scale provide detailed instructions for assessing and scoring patients; for example:

> Doing personal toilet: 5 = patient can wash hands and face, comb hair, clean teeth, and shave. He may use any kind of razor but must put in blade or plug in razor without help as well as get it from drawer or cabinet. Female patients must put on own make-up, if used, but need not braid or style hair.

The scores are intended to reflect the amount of time and assistance a patient requires. However, the scoring method is inconsistent in that changes by a given number of points do not reflect equivalent changes in disability across different activities.

Moreover, as its authors point out, the scale is restricted in that changes can occur beyond the end points of the scale. The scale is also limited to physical activities and does not take mental status or social well-being into account. It is restricted to measuring one aspect of quality of life.

Validity

The problem with such observed assessments is that they do not necessarily reflect what the person usually does in everyday life. There have been a number of studies reporting predictive validity for the Barthel Index. The Barthel Index has been shown to be capable of successfully predicting mortality among stroke patients, length of hospital stay and progress as independently rated by a physician (Wylie and White 1964). Evidence of its correlational validity with other scales comes mainly from studies comparing it with the PULSES profile, which give correlations of −0.74 to −0.90 (Granger *et al.* 1979).

Reliability

Granger *et al.* (1979) reported a test-retest reliability of 0.89 with severely disabled adults, and an inter-rater agreement exceeding 0.95. Although it is a popular scale among clinicians worldwide, further evidence of its reliability is required.

In sum, while simplicity is an attraction of the scale, it also poses a major limitation on its use. Further testing is required before its use can be recommended for widespread use in community surveys and evaluations. Despite its acknowledged limitations, there is an increasing body of literature supporting its use with specific groups of patients such as those with neurological disability (Collin *et al*; 1988; Wade and Collin 1988).

The Quality of Well-Being Scale (QWBS)

The Quality of Well-Being Scale was developed to operationalize 'wellness' for a general health-policy model. This was an attempt to develop an alternative to economic cost-benefit analysis for resource allocation, for example, by comparing the health status of groups of individuals for the evaluation of health-care programmes (Kaplan *et al.* 1976; Bush 1984).

It can be used with general populations and applied to any type of disease. The items in the interview schedule were drawn mainly from the USA Health Interview Survey and from the Social Security Administration Survey, but the schedule has been extensively tested on large groups of nurses and graduate students and revised. The QWBS combines mortality with estimates of the quality of life. The scale quantifies the health output of a treatment in terms of years of life, adjusted for their diminished quality, that it is responsible for. It is based on a three-component model of health. First, the assessment of health begins with an assessment of function status, based on the individual's performance. The authors listed all the ways by which a disease or injury can affect a person's behaviour and performance (Kaplan *et al.* 1976). Second, a value reflecting the relative desirability (utility) is assigned to each functional level (Fanshel and Bush 1970).

Responses to a branching questionnaire are used to assign subjects to one of a number of discrete function states. It is based on a model of health which encompasses symptom/problem, mobility, physical activity and social activity. The QWBS has been used in many evaluative studies of pulmonary disease and in drug trials (Toevs *et al.* 1984; Bombardier *et al.* 1986). Several areas of application have been reported by Bush (1984), most of which are unpublished. The scale includes death. This avoids the problem inherent in other indices where, as death is frequently ignored, the death of a disabled person appears to improve the population estimate of health status. Third, information is also collected about future changes (prognosis). This permits a distinction between two people with equal functional disability but one of whom is terminally ill.

The interview schedule is long, and a 30-page manual is purchasable from the authors. The questionnaire takes 10–15 minutes to administer. The QWB is administered by trained interviewers. It can be administered to proxies where people are not able to reply (e.g. stroke victims).

Content

The Quality of Well-Being Scale consists of three ordinal scales on dimensions of daily activity. Combinations of each of the three scales of mobility, physical and social activity were initially taken to define 29 function levels. Subsequent modification has increased the number of function levels to 43. Each function level can be linked with a separate classification of symptoms and problems. Questions are based on performance, not capacity. Four aspects of function are covered, mobility/confinement, physical activity, social activity (e.g. work, housekeeping) and self-care. The categories on each scale range from full independence to death. The physical ability scale has four categories and the others have five.

Respondents are given a list of 22 'symptom/problem' complexes and asked to identify all that applied to them during the preceding six days. They are then asked to indicate which of these has 'bothered them most'. Next, they are asked about mobility, physical and social activity. Actual ability rather than capacity to perform is asked about. Examples of the scale items are:

Mobility	*Physical activity*	*Social activity*
Drove car and used bus or train	Walked without physical problems	Did work, school, or housework and other activities
Did not drive or had help to use bus or train	Walked with physical limitations	Limited in amount or kind of work, school or housework

Scoring

Respondents' functional status is classified for each day on the scales of mobility, physical and social activity. The QWBS score is calculated by combining this information with the symptom/problem responses, using a set of preference weights. The latter were developed on the basis of interviews with 800 respondents in a household survey in which respondents were asked to rate different health states on a ten-point scale ranging from death to perfect health. The ratings were used in a multiple regression analysis to obtain weights for different responses. Scores are calculated separately for each of the six days, and the QWBS score is expressed as the average of these. The final score ranges from 0 (equated with death) to 1 (perfect health) (Patrick *et al.* 1973a; 1973b). For each of the 43 function levels a 'preference weight' has been established empirically, ranging from 1 (complete well-being) to 0 (death). The appropriate preference weight is assigned to the respondents' functional-ability level, and the resulting score is known as the Quality of Well-Being score. The authors noted that it is possible to provide a score below zero to represent a state 'worse than death' (Kaplan and Bush 1982). The weights assigned represent preferences of the relative importance that 67 subjects or members of society assigned to each functional level. The third stage of rating involves adjusting for prognosis (Kaplan *et al* 1976; 1979). Further testing for the validation of the scaling technique has been reported by Kaplan and Ernst (1983). The means and variances of preferences for attributes of quality of life did not change over time (Kaplan *et al.* 1978).

Validity

The content validity of the QWBS has been stated by Kaplan *et al.* (1976). Its content validity as an index of disability is enhanced by incorporating death. Kaplan *et al.* (1976) report correlations of −0.75 between the QWBS and number of reported symptoms, and of 0.96 between the QWBS and the number of chronic health problems. The correlation between the QWBS and the number of physician contacts in the preceding eight days was 0.55. It correlates well (0.76) with self-rated quality of life. Thus it is said by its authors to have convergent validity. Its predictive value has been reported to be between 0.95 and 0.98 and sensitivity at 0.90, on the basis of data from 1,324 subjects with a range of diseases and injuries. It is able to discriminate between changes in life quality over time (Kaplan *et al.* 1976).

The Quality of Well-Being Scale was used by Leighton Read *et al.* (1987) in a study of 400 out-patients in Boston, Massachusetts, USA. The authors tested this scale, the SIP and the Rand Corporation's General Health Rating Index (GHRI) for convergent-construct validity, content and discriminant validity. The findings for convergent-construct validity were similar to those achieved by the developers of the scales – the correlations between scales was moderately high (0.46–0.55). They reported the GHRI to be the easiest to use, as they found both the SIP and the QWB scales required a major commitment to interviewer training. All were equally acceptable to respondents. The QWBS contained more items than the others on specific symptoms; in contrast the SIP contained more detail on dysfunction. The authors concluded that each scale was a valid measure of health status.

Reliability

The reliability coefficient obtained when judges reassessed scale values for 29 function levels was 0.90 (Kaplan and Bush 1982). Test-retest reliability is between 0.93 and 0.98 (Kaplan et al. 1978; Bush 1984). The internal-consistency reliability estimates for the QWBS overall score have been reported for four populations and reliability estimates have exceeded 0.90. The scale is sufficiently reliable for use in making group comparisons.

While the QWBS is advantageous in that it incorporates mortality, its main disadvantages are its complexity, and the requirement that it needs to be administered by trained interviewers.

The Crichton Royal Behaviour Rating Scale (CRBRS)

The Crichton Royal Behaviour Rating Scale was developed by Robinson (1968) and refined and tested for reliability and validity by Wilkin and Jolley (1979), on the basis of samples of people in residential homes for the elderly, geriatric and psychiatric wards. The scale has had a wide application in the UK and was used for the evaluation of Department of Health and district health authority-funded nursing homes (Bond et al. 1989; Bowling and Formby 1990) and for the assessment of residential care of the elderly (Willcocks et al. 1987).

The CRBRS was designed for use with elderly people living in institutions. It is completed by a third person who knows the respondent well (e.g. a nurse in a hospital ward would complete it on behalf of a patient known well to him/her). The modified CRBRS contains ten items, five relating to functional ability (mobility, feeding, dressing, bathing, continence) and five relate to mental disturbance (memory, orientation, communication, co-operation, restlessness). The confusion sub-scale can be used independently of the functional-ability scale.

As the scale was designed for use with populations resident in institutions, home-care activities were excluded. Although the research reports containing evidence of the scale's reliability and validity are now out of print, a brief description of the scale has been published by Wilkin and Thompson (1989). Interviewer training is required.

Notes of guidance are provided for interviewers to elicit the appropriate questions. The interviewer is expected to probe and ask for examples of behaviour before a classification is made. The emphasis of the scale is on behaviour (what the person actually does), rather than on ability. A set of structured questions has been designed by Bond *et al.* (1989) for use with the interviewers' assessments, with high correlations between the two. The interviewer assessment without the structured questions takes approximately three minutes, the assessment with the structured questions can extend the interview to seven to ten minutes (Wilkin and Thompson 1989; Bowling and Formby 1990).

Content

Examples of the rating scale are:

Dressing
0 Correct
1 Imperfect but adequate
2 Adequate with minimum of supervision
3 Inadequate unless continually supervised
4 Unable to dress or to retain clothing

Feeding
0 Correct unaided at appropriate times
1 Adequate with minimum of supervision
2 Inadequate unless constantly supervised
3 Requires feeding

Memory
0 Complete
1 Occasionally forgetful
2 Short-term loss
3 Short- and long-term loss

Orientation
0 Complete
1 Oriented in ward, identifies people correctly
2 Misidentifies but can find way about
3 Cannot find way to bed or toilet without assistance
4 Completely lost

Full details of the CRBRS, together with the full-scale items, interviewer notes and structured questions designed by Bond *et al.* (1989) to accompany the rating scale, are reproduced by Wilkin and Thompson (1989).

Scoring

Each item is scored 0 to 4, except memory and feeding which are scored 0 to 3; thus these two items were designed to make a smaller contribution to the overall score. Individual items are added to obtain the total score. These are grouped into six ranges, although the authors state that they do not represent levels of dependency: 0–1, 2–5, 6–10, 11–15, 16–20, 21–38. It is unclear what the different scale scores represent.

A sub-scale for confusion can also be derived, consisting of the items relating to memory, orientation and communication. These sub-scale scores are totalled and grouped into four ranges: 0–1 (lucid); 2–3 (intermediate); 4–6 (moderately confused); 7–11 (severely confused) (Evans *et al.* 1981).

Validity

Thompson (1984) used factor analysis to assess the construct validity of the CRBRS. She reported that the ten items reflected two dimensions of dependency: capacity for self-care and ability to walk.

The research reports with details of testing for validity and reliability are out of print, but Wilkin and Thompson (1989) have summarized the results. They reported that total scale scores of 10 or more were associated with a diagnosis of psychiatric disorder. The study reported by Evans *et al.* (1981) suggested that confusion sub-scale scores of 4 or more were associated with a clinical diagnosis of dementia. Total scale scores and the confusion sub-scale scores have been compared with independent clinical assessments and the modified Roth-Hopkins mental-state test (the correlations for the latter range between 0.75 and 0.82) (Vardon and Blessed 1986; Wilkin and Thompson 1989). There has been little work testing the validity of the CRBRS.

Wilkin and Thompson (1989) caution that the scale is insufficiently sensitive as a tool for assessing change over time and should be used to provide population profiles. The problem with using the scale to assess individual change over time is that reliance on different informants to complete the scale may produce bias.

Reliability

The emphasis of the scale on behaviour rather than ability in theory minimizes problems with reliability. In practice, however, it is likely that ratings will reflect the philosophy of the institution; for example, staff working in institutions which encourage independence are likely to assess patients/residents as less dependent than staff in institutions which encourage dependency.

Thompson (1984) assessed the internal reliability of the capacity for self-care dimension of the scale. She reported that reliability can be increased by removing the items relating to feeding, restlessness and co-operation, and by treating mobility as a separate dimension. Wilkin and Jolley (1979) examined inter-rater reliability, using two interviewers to assess the same informant; the correlations obtained were greater than 0.90. Far more testing for reliability is required.

There are some difficulties within the scale which have not yet been resolved; for example, the classification of ability to use stairs in the case of a respondent who lives on the ground floor and does not need to use stairs.

Despite the limited evidence about its reliability and validity, the CRBRS is popular in the UK as a measure of functioning for use with elderly people living in institutions. It is fairly concise and easily administered by a trained interviewer. Its popularity in this area is probably partly due to the advantage it has in being specifically designed for use with a third party.

The Clifton Assessment Procedures for the Elderly (CAPE)

The Clifton Assessment Procedures for the Elderly is the most extensively tested measure of dependency in widespread use in the UK, particularly in relation to psychological assessments of the elderly. It was developed for use with elderly people living in institutions, and tested for validity by Pattie and Gilleard (1979). A manual is available which provides details of use and also normative data for a range of patient populations (Pattie and Gilleard 1979). The CAPE consists of two schedules, designed to measure behaviour and cognitive performance, known as the Behaviour and the Cognitive Assessment Scale. The Cognitive Assessment Scale was originally known as the Clifton Assessment Scale, and can be completed by an elderly person in five to fifteen minutes. The Behaviour Rating Scale is a short version of the Stockton Geriatric Rating Scale, designed for use with elderly people in hospital. The whole test can take between five to thirty minutes, depending on the mental and functional ability of the respondent. It is designed to be completed by a third party who knows the respondent well. Interviewer training is necessary.

Content

The Cognitive Performance Scale consists of a battery of tests which includes items such as the person tracing a circular route with a pencil, avoiding obstacles; the information/orientation items include the usual memory tests of own place of residence, name of the prime minister, date, etc., and, more unusually, knowledge of the colours of the British flag.

The Behavioural Rating Scale contains 18 items. Four items relate to mobility, continence and activities of daily living. The remaining items relate to confused behaviour. The scale asks about current-level functioning. The scale focuses heavily on the behavioural problems of those elderly people who are mentally infirm. The rater is instructed to rate people according to their level of current functioning, and to take into account behaviour over the past two weeks.

The authors suggest that the CAPE relates to four sub-scales: physical disability, apathy, communication difficulties and social disturbance. Examples of the behaviour-rating scale are:

When bathing or dressing, he/she requires:

0 No assistance
1 Some assistance
2 Maximum assistance

With regard to walking, he/she:

0 Shows no signs of weakness
1 Walks slowly without aid, or uses a stick
2 Is unable to walk, or if able to walk, needs frame, crutches or someone by his/her side

He/she is confused (unable to find way around, loses possessions, etc.):

0 Almost never confused
1 Sometimes confused
2 Almost always confused

His/her sleep pattern at night is:

0 Almost never awake
1 Sometimes awake
2 Often awake

Scoring

The 18 items are added to form a total score, or selected items are added to produce sub-scale scores. Each item has a range of scores from 0 (no/few problems) to 2 (frequent/constant problems). Four sub-scales can be created from the items relating to physical disability, apathy, communication difficulties and social disturbance. The total scale range of scores is from 0 to 36. A score of 0–3 indicates independence; 4–7 indicates low dependency; 8–12 indicates medium dependency; 13–17 indicates high dependency and 18–36 is maximum dependency. No item weights are used.

Validity

Early versions of the scale were shown to correlate with clinicians' assessments about appropriate levels of care for females but not males. The sample size was small, 38. The authors also report correlations with other scales such as the Wechsler Memory Scale, but sample sizes were too small to be conclusive. This provides weak evidence of the scale's concurrent validity (Smith *et al.* 1981).

Black *et al.* (1990) compared the diagnostic ability of the CAPE, in relation to dementia, with the diagnosis made by the computer program AGECAT and a clinical diagnosis made by a psychiatrist. The sample was an elderly sample of patients from a general practice (112 were selected from 378 who had been tested three years previously when aged 70+ using a 13-item mental-function test). The authors reported that the sensitivity of the CAPE was low, probably because it identified only the more severe cases. The CAPE only detected about half the number of known cases.

In relation to behaviour, Pattie and Gilleard (1979) have reported that the CAPE can discriminate between elderly people requiring differing degrees of help, with different levels of social adjustment following admission to a residential home, and between mentally infirm people who survive and those who die.

Results of factor analyses showed that two factor structures emerged for three groups of elderly people tested, and no clear factor structure emerged for non-psychiatrically ill elderly people (Pattie and Gilleard 1979). The four sub-scales suggested by the authors for analysing the Behaviour Rating Scale data were not supported. Factor analyses carried out on the CAPE by Twining and Allen (1981), on the basis of 903 people in residential homes for the elderly, also failed to support the four suggested sub-scales.

Reliability

Pattie and Gilleard (1979) report inter-item correlations, and all are fairly high. This suggests that items are consistent and are measuring the same dimensions of dependency. Inter-rater reliability for the four sub-scales was tested on psychiatric and psychogeriatric patients and people in residential homes for the elderly; the correlations were all 0.70 or higher with the exception of the correlation for 'communication difficulties' which was low. Tests for inter-rater reliability for the total scale showed wide variations. Smith *et al.* (1981), in their study of 38 elderly mentally handicapped patients, reported inter-rater a reliability coefficient of 0.58 between two nursing sisters.

Test-retest reliability coefficients range from 0.56 to 0.90 at retests over two to three days with 38 hospital patients aged 65 and over, and at retests over two to three months. The six month test-retest reliabilities, based on 39 new admissions to homes for the elderly range from 0.69 to 0.84 (Pattie and Gilleard 1979).

Although this dependency scale has undergone more testing than the Crichton Royal Behaviour Rating Scale, evidence is still limited and for reliability it is weak. The scale, along with others in common use in the UK, has been reviewed by Wilkin and Thompson (1989). They draw attention to ambiguities in the scale wording, for example the terms 'sometimes' and 'frequently' are not defined and therefore likely to be interpreted differently by different raters. The scale has also been reviewed by Mulgrave (1985) who reported its main advantages as being short and easily administered, although further evidence of its reliability and validity is required.

4
Broader measures of health status

Broader measures of health status generally focus on individuals' subjective perceptions of their health. Subjective or perceived health may be defined as an individual's experience of mental, physical and social events as they impinge upon feelings of well-being (Hunt 1988). Many studies in medical sociology have indicated the importance of the perceptual component of illness in determining whether people feel ill or whether they seek help.

While many scales of broader-health status exist and are to be preferred to single-item questions, a popular single-item measure on both sides of the Atlantic consists of asking respondents to rate their health as 'excellent, good, fair or poor'. Some researchers ask respondents to rate this in relation to their age (e.g. Cartwright and Anderson 1981). This single-item measure of self-perceived health status has been found to be related to eventual mortality and to rates of recovery from episodes of ill health (National Heart and Lung Institute 1976; Singer et al. 1976). Mortality has been found to be two to three times greater for people who report their health as poor than for those who rate their health as excellent (Kaplan and Camacho 1983). Perceived health has been found to be more closely related to use of health services than medical condition (Goldstein et al. 1984). Although the ratings on this question correlate well with subsequent mortality and admission to hospital, it has been subjected to three main criticisms, it provides no information about why people rate themselves as 'good', 'fair', 'excellent' or 'poor'. Also, it provides only four response choices and around half of a general population sample may rate themselves as in 'excellent' or 'good' health (Bowling and Cartwright 1982; Ware 1984). This measure may be contextual and vary over time with people's varying expectations. Self-ratings of health are often criticized as subjective, but their subjectivity is their strength because they reflect personal evaluations of health.

Given that subjectivity is a major criticism levelled at this type of indicator, it merits some discussion. Health indicators have largely been developed within the era of science based on the logical positivist paradigm. This inevitably leads to suspicion when data are presented which are based on subjective experience. This is despite the research questioning the reliability of 'objective' data. The concordance rate of clinical and pathological diagnoses has been shown to be as low as 45.3 per cent (Heasman and Lipworth 1966), and several studies have reported on the arbitrary nature of normal values in biochemistry (Grasbeck and Saris 1969; Bradwell et al. 1974), and of the problem of establishing a dividing line between sick and healthy in relation to diabetes, hypertension and glaucoma (Cochrane and Holland 1971). One Swedish out-patient study also found that there was only 50 per cent agreement between doctors and patients on whether treatment had been successful (Orth-Gomer et al. 1979). Similar results have been obtained in relation to low back pain and outcome of surgery, blood-pressure treatment, and results of surgery for peptic ulcer (Hall et al. 1976; Thomas and Lyttle 1980, Jachuck et al. 1982).

Other measurement formats which are commonly used in studies of health status are symptom check-lists. These also have their limitations, but are generally considered to be useful tools if used in conjunction with scaled measurement techniques. There are numerous examples of check-lists of symptoms presented to respondents in surveys. Respondents are typically asked to indicate which, if any, they currently suffer from. George and Bearon (1980) give some examples of symptom check-lists; other examples can be found in Cartwright's national surveys in the UK (e.g. Dunnell and Cartwright 1972; Cartwright and Anderson 1981; Bowling and Cartwright 1982), and in the Rand Health Insurance Study Questionnaires (Stewart et al. 1978). Diagnostic data obtained in population surveys are neither specific nor precise. Questions that ask about symptoms produce a high proportion of affirmative responses (e.g. Dunnell and Cartwright 1972). Items focusing on trivial problems are unlikely to have much discriminatory power in terms of monitoring change between groups over time. They may include not only response errors, but diagnostic errors – many people do not know the specific nature nor cause of their afflictions. Reporting of morbidity may also depend on tolerance levels and pain thresholds; the decision to restrict activities reflects the individual's attitude towards illness and self-care, the expectations and demands of others (family, employer, friends), knowledge and under-standing of symptoms experienced and other social and cultural factors.

There is a fundamental question that remains unanswered with measures of health status which should be noted at this point: why are people with poor mental health (e.g. depression) more likely to rate their health status, functional ability and social support as low? In some cases poor mental health will distort perceptions of health and well-being, and poor physical health can also lead to poor mental health and well-being (including reduced social interaction). Researchers need to be aware of this problem, which leads to difficulties in interpreting results.

Given that a subjective measure of health status is required, and it is accepted that single-item measures are limited in value, the issue becomes that of which measure to choose. The researcher also has to decide whether a general and/or specific measure is required, depending on the nature of the study. There is little point in including a health measure if it is unlikely to detect the effects of the treatment or symptoms specific to the condition. Some specific disease-related scales do exist, although the Nottingham Health Profile and the Sickness Impact Profile have also been used as more general measures of quality of life and are apparently successful at distinguishing between patient types.

The case for using general, rather than specific, indicators of health status in population surveys has been clearly argued by Kaplan (1988). For example, detailed information about specific disease categories may appear overwhelming to many respondents not suffering from them. Also the use of disease-specific measures precludes the possibility of comparing programmes (e.g. health promotion) that are directed at different groups suffering from different diseases. Policy analysis requires a general measure of health status. Broader measures of physical, social and psychological functioning exist, but their use in the UK has been limited. If necessary, as in the case of a study of a specific disease group, global measures can be supplemented with disease-effect questions.

The following sections describe the most well-known and best tested measures of broader-health status that are currently available. All were developed in the USA, except the Nottingham Health Profile, and the Functional Limitations Profile (an adaptation of the Sickness Impact Profile) both of which were developed in the UK.

The Sickness Impact Profile (SIP)

One of the best instruments developed in the USA has been the Sickness Impact Profile (SIP) (Deyo *et al.* 1982; 1983). The Sickness Impact Profile was developed as a measure of perceived health status, for use as an outcome measure for health-care evaluation across a wide range of health problems and diseases, across demographic and cultural groups. Sickness is measured in relation to its impact on behaviour. The profile emphasizes sickness-related dysfunction rather than disease. It was designed to be sensitive to differences in health status in terms of minor morbidity (Bergner *et al.* 1976a; 1976b; Bergner *et al.* 1981; Gilson *et al.* 1979).

The Sickness Impact Profile concentrates on assessing the impact of sickness on daily activities and behaviour, rather than feelings and clinical reports. The justification was that feelings are difficult to measure and subjective and thus difficult to validate, and clinical reports can be provided only where someone has sought medical care. The authors felt that behavioural reports were less subject to bias than feelings, although reported behaviour can be influenced by perceptual bias and behaviour can be influenced by feelings. The authors acknowledged that the SIP does not measure positive functioning.

The SIP was developed on the basis of a literature review and after extracting statements from health professionals, healthy and ill lay people which described 'sickness related behaviour dysfunction' (Bergner et al. 1981).

The populations and patient groups involved in its development varied widely and included in-patients, out-patients, and home-care patients with chronic diseases, patients in intensive care units, patients undergoing hip replacements and arthritis patients. It may be self- or interviewer-administered. It takes 20–30 minutes to complete. Deyo et al. (1983) recognized the problem of its length and suggested that attempts to shorten it might augment patient acceptability. A sub-sample of the participants in their study were asked about their opinions of the SIP and, while most said it was acceptable, the few complaints elicited concerned its length and the fact that it was not disease specific. The authors suggest that the sub-scales could be used independently if desired (e.g. the physical function sub-scale consists of only 45 of the 136 items). A study asking interviewers to make ratings of the ease of application of the SIP by Read et al. (1987) found that the length of the SIP was reported to be tedious, largely because of the repetition contained. They also reported that the SIP involved a major commitment to interviewer training time (at least a week). More optimistic findings were reported by Hall et al. (1987). The SIP was used in a general study of patient outcome based in a general practice setting in Sydney, Australia by Hall et al. (1987). The SIP was used along with the General Health Questionnaire (see page 108) and the Rand Health-Insurance Battery; 160 questionnaires were completed by patients, and only 3 per cent did not complete all the questions across the three scales.

There have been many applications of the SIP to a wide range of patient groups, mainly in the USA, but also in the UK and other parts of the world. A recent application in the UK was by Fletcher et al. (1988) in a randomized controlled trial of outcome of drug treatment of angina patients. The SIP has been widely used in the US heart-transplantation evaluations. Many applications of the SIP have been described by Wenger et al. (1984). The advantage this wide application provides is that scores for many population groups are available for comparison.

Content

The SIP incorporates questions, not only on functioning, but also on feelings of emotional well-being and social functioning. This contains 136 items referring to illness-related dysfunction in 12 areas: work, recreation, emotion, affect, home life, sleep, rest, eating, ambulation, mobility, communication and social interaction. A typical set of questions from the SIP requests respondents to tick statements which apply to them on a given day and are related to their state of health:

I spend much of the day lying down in order to rest.
I sit during much of the day.
I am sleeping or dozing most of the time – day and night.
I stand up only with someone's help.
I kneel, stoop, or bend down only by holding on to something.
I am in a restricted position all the time.
I do work around the house only for short periods of time or rest often.
I am doing less of the regular daily work around the house that I would usually do.
I am not doing any of the house cleaning that I would usually do.
I am going out less to visit people.
I am not going out to visit people at all.
I am doing fewer social activities with groups of people.

Only those questions to which the respondents answers 'yes' are recorded; thus there is no way of knowing in the analysis whether the columns left blank represent 'no' replies or whether the respondent/interviewer omitted them deliberately or in error.

Scoring

The responses to the 136 items can be summarized by component, by physical or psychosocial dimension or as a single score with a range of 0–100. The lower the score the better the respondents' health status.

The score for the SIP may be calculated using item weights that indicate the relative severity of limitation implied by each statement. The weights were derived from equal-appearing interval-scaling procedures involving more than 100 judges. The judges rated each item on an equal-interval 11-point scale from 'minimally dysfunctional' to 'severely dysfunctional'. The scaling technique has been justified and described by Carter et al. (1976).

The overall score for the SIP is calculated by adding the scale values for each item checked across all categories and dividing by the maximum possible dysfunction score for the SIP. This figure is then multiplied by 100 to obtain the SIP overall score. The two sub-scores (physical and psychosocial) are calculated using a similar formula but limiting the calculations to the relevant items.

Although the many studies using the SIP have ensured the existence of scores for comparison, it is unclear what each score represents. Many other scales also suffer this problem (e.g. the HAQ). It is known that a normal population may score only 2 or 3 on the SIP, increasing to the mid-30s for terminally ill cancer and stroke patients, but the precise definition of scale points has not so far been tackled.

The study based in Sydney, Australia by Hall *et al.* (1987) reported that results were skewed towards the healthy end of the SIP scale. Eighteen per cent of patients scored zero on all components. There were no scores above 25 (range of possible scores 0–100). This pattern was repeated within components.

Validity

The early validation studies of the SIP tested it against self-assessments of health status, clinicians' assessments of health status and functional assessment instruments; 278 people were assessed. SIP scores discriminated between four sub-groups divided according to severity of sickness, and correlations between measures were better for patients' self-assessments than physicians' assessments (0.69 with a self-assessment of limitation; 0.63 with a self-assessment of sickness; 0.50 with a clinician's assessment of limitation; and 0.40 with a clinician's assessment of sickness). The combined SIP score was tested against the Katz ADL scale with a correlation of 0.64; and the correlation between the SIP and the National Health Interview Survey Instrument was 0.55 (Bergner *et al.* 1981).

Convergent and discriminant validity was evaluated using the multi-trait–multi-method technique. Clinical validity was assessed by comparing clinical judgements with SIP scores; all achieved good results. These have been described in some detail by Bergner *et al.* (1981). More recent evidence pointing to its strong validity properties has been provided by Read *et al.* (1987).

The Australian study by Hall *et al.* (1987) reported that, with the use of a correlation threshold of –0.30, the SIP correlated with the Rand index. The Rand mental-health index correlated with the SIP items relating to social interaction, emotional behaviour and alertness; and ambulation from the SIP correlated with the Rand physical-abilities scale. Home-management and social-interaction items from the SIP correlated with the role-functioning items on the Rand battery. However, the correlations ranged from 0.32 to 0.54.

The Sickness Impact Profile has been used successfully in clinical trials (Bergner *et al.* 1976a; 1976b; 1981), is sensitive to change, is valuable for assessing the impact of illness on the chronically ill and for measuring the effects of non-curative interventions. It has been used in a randomized controlled trial of early exercise and counselling for patients with myocardial infarction. This study reported that the SIP showed that the group undergoing exercise plus counselling reported better functioning (Ott *et al.* 1983). It has also been used to evaluate treatment for patients with end-stage renal disease, with the result that transplantation patients had better SIP scores (Hart and Evans 1987).

More negative results relating to sensitivity were reported by Hall *et al.* (1987) who tested the SIP against the Rand Health Insurance Study batteries. The Rand and the SIP were reported to be measuring different aspects of health. The range of scores for the Rand measures was less skewed than for the SIP. The problem with an instrument which registers high scores is that it may be unable to measure improvements in health. Thus the Rand measures have better discriminative abilities than the SIP.

Reliability

Work began on the SIP in 1972, and tests for reliability and validity continued to be conducted by its authors for over a decade. Patients studied included those with hypothyroidism, rheumatoid arthritis and hip replacements. The details of the reliability tests conducted on the SIP are reported by Bergner *et al.* (1981). Earlier reliability tests on SIPs of differing lengths before the development of the 136 version are reported by Pollard *et al.* (1976; 1978).

Test-retest reliability was high (0.88–0.92). Internal consistency was also high (0.81–0.97). The interviewer-administered versions scored better in each case than mailed or self-completed versions. Deyo *et al.* (1983) applied the SIP to 79 patients with arthritis and found that test-retest reliability for 23 patients tested was 0.91. It was found to have better reliability than the traditional functional scales of the American Rheumatism Association and patients' self-ratings of function. Test-retest reliability was better for the overall score than for each of the dimensions.

UK adaptations

Although patient acceptance of the SIP was judged by the US authors to be good, it has been rejected for use in evaluations of heart-disease treatment programmes in the UK on the grounds of its length, and the more concise Nottingham Health Profile selected in preference (Buxton 1983; O'Brien 1988).

A modified version of the SIP has been developed at St Thomas's Hospital, London, for a community disability survey. The modified version is called the Functional Limitations Profile (FLP) (Patrick 1982). Linguistic changes were made and scale weights were recalculated, although these agreed closely with the original weights of the USA version. The translation has been criticized by Hunt *et al.* (1986) on the grounds that language changes alone do not satisfy the requirements for cross-cultural adaptations. The changes made are fairly minimal and the FLP is still 136 items long, is designed to be interviewer-administered and contains the same range of scores from 0 (low) to 100 (high), although the weighting is different.

The authors later reported that FLP and SIP items grouped satisfactorily into five global measures: physical, psychosocial, eating, communication and work. They found the items related to age and number of medical conditions but were poor predictors of service use (Charlton *et al.* 1983).

A UK application of the Functional Limitations Profile was a study of 92 patients with chronic obstructive pulmonary disease by Williams and Bury (1989) who reported good correlations between the FLP and clinical data.

Another application of the FLP has been reported by Fitzpatrick *et al.* (1988) in their study of 105 patients with rheumatoid arthritis assessed over a 15-month period. They used both the FLP and the HAQ, but reported only modest levels of sensitivity and specificity in relation to data on clinical change for each. Although the authors acknowledged that the SIP provided more information and was more precise than the short HAQ, they caution that this has to be weighed against the simpler measurement assumptions and shorter time required to administer the HAQ.

The conclusion relating to the FLP is that it requires far more testing for reliability and validity before it can be considered the UK alternative to the SIP.

Vetter *et al.* (1989) used their own adaptation of the SIP along with the Barthel Index to assess rehabilitation outcomes among a pilot sample of 59 elderly people receiving either home or day hospital care in Wales. The authors substantially changed the style of the SIP. They reported that respondents found the 'I' format (e.g. 'I dress myself, but do so very slowly') confusing. They became confused about who the 'I' was referring to. The statements were therefore changed to actual questions (e.g. 'Do you dress yourself, but do so very slowly?').

A further problem found with the use of the SIP by these UK researchers was that some questions were not applicable to all patients. Thus the question 'Are you unable to walk up and down hills?' in the original profile could be answered only 'yes' or 'no'. The researchers thus added a 'not applicable' category to avoid confusion, for example, for those who were bed/chairfast. The physical dimension scale of the SIP was found to have acceptable validity and was judged as a suitable measure of outcome (other dimensions are yet to be tested), although the correlations were unreported. The SIP was also found to be a stable measure when repeated eight weeks later on the patients (they were not expected to change in relation to physical state).

The advantages of the SIP and its adaptations are that it can be self-administered or interview based, it can be used with chronically or acutely ill patients, it has been adapted for use in the UK as the Functional Limitations Profile, it is sensitive to change, and it is well tested for reliability and validity. Given its excellent properties of reliability and validity, it has been highly recommended for use as a gold standard by McDowell and Newell (1987) in their review of health status measures. Its limitations are its length and it can be used only with people who are regarded or who regard themselves as ill.

The Nottingham Health Profile (NHP)

The Nottingham Health Profile was developed in the UK and is based on lay perceptions of health status. The conceptual basis of the NHP was that it should reflect lay rather than professional definitions of health. It was developed after interviews with a large number of lay people about the effects of illness on behaviour. Hunt *et al.* (1986) commented that their pilot interviewing to develop the NHP demonstrated that lay people had a limited range of language for describing good health and well-being which would have made the creation of a comprehensive health index difficult. The NHP is not an index of disease, illness or disability but relates rather to how people feel when they are experiencing various states of ill health. As a survey tool it is useful in assessing whether people have a (severe) health problem at all, but diagnostic data would be required to point to the kind of health problem. Similarly, it does not attempt to be a comprehensive measure of health related quality of life. It is too short to assess the impact of a condition on quality of life. For this, combinations of measures are required: a functional-disability scale, symptom and pain indices, a measure of psychological disturbance, quantitative and more qualitative methods of the impact on social functioning (e.g. work, interpersonal relationships and social support, domestic life, etc.). The NHP can provide only a shallow profile of effects on these aspects.

Pilot work with the NHP led to the identification of relevant concepts. Statements were drawn which exemplified those concepts and, after further piloting, statements were finally categorized into six areas: physical mobility, pain, sleep, energy, emotional reactions and social isolation. The Nottingham Health Profile is designed for self-completion, is concise and easily administered and is the only measure of perceived health which has been extensively tested and developed for use in Europe.

Hunt *et al.* (1986) reported that, when the NHP is based on a postal survey, people are unlikely to return it if they have a high number of zero scores (no problems). People felt they had nothing to contribute to the study. Pilot work has been undertaken with positive items as dummies: 'I sleep soundly at night'; 'I am usually free of any pain'.

In the UK the Nottingham Health Profile has been used to evaluate the outcome of many therapies from the patient's perspective, and to assess the perceived health status of patients before and after undergoing specific surgery (e.g. coronary bypass, varicose veins, haemorrhoids, heart transplantation and various orthopaedic conditions).

The NHP is short and simple, and it can be used with groups of patients or a general population. Although it is suitable for people who are not necessarily unhealthy or ill, like many others it focuses on negative rather than positive experiences. Population norms exist for the instrument, as do scores on individual patient groups (Hunt *et al.* 1984).

Content

Part I measures perceived or subjective health status by asking for yes/no responses to 38 simple statements of six dimensions: mobility, pain, energy, sleep, emotional reactions and social isolation. Each dimension has a range of possible scores of 0–100.

Part II asks about any effects of health on seven areas of daily life: work, looking after the home, social life, home life, sex life, interests, hobbies and holidays. Part II items are coded 1 for 'yes' and 0 for 'no' and then scored. Part II is not always a useful addition. For some groups several items do not apply, e.g. the elderly, the unemployed, the disabled, those on low incomes. The authors have recently carried out developmental work on Part II and recommend that Part II is not used until this has been completed; full details are available from them.

Examples of the NHP items include:

Part I

This asks about the applicability of statements to the respondent at the present time:

I'm tired all the time.
I have pain at night.
Things are getting me down.
I have unbearable pain.
I take tablets to help me sleep.

Part II

Is your present state of health causing problems with your:

Job of work?
Looking after the home?
Social life?
Home life?

A main advantage of the NHP is that its authors have published a book containing a review of the development of the scale, studies of its reliability and validity, the NHP items and a users' manual (Hunt *et al.* 1986).

Scoring

The NHP is scored with scores ranging from 0 (no problems) to 100 (where all problems in a section are affirmed). It has been extensively tested for reliability and validity, and results have been good.

The weights for the NHP were derived using Thurstone's method of paired comparisons. Judgements were obtained from several hundred people and converted into weights using the appropriate formula (McKenna *et al.* 1981).

The NHP scores are not 'true' numbers but are obtained from a scaling technique; thus the appropriate statistical tests for testing hypotheses are non-parametric. Its highly skewed distribution of scores (see page 67) means that careful consideration needs to be given to the application of statistical tests as many assume that the results are normally distributed; although statistical transformations can be applied to skewed data, thus permitting the application of parametric statistics.

Part I of the NHP requires respondents to indicate 'yes' or 'no' according to whether the statement applies to them 'in general at the present time'. Relative weights are applied to these. All statements relate to limitations on activity or aspects of distress. Dimension scores of 100 indicate the presence of all limitations listed, and a zero score the absence of limitations, but these two extremes do not reflect the extremes of death or perfect health.

Part II relates to seven areas of task performance affected by health (page 65). Respondents answer 'yes' if their present state of health is causing problems with the activity. Part II has no weights: a count of affirmative responses is used as a summary statistic.

It is not possible to calculate an overall health status score, although aggregation within categories is permitted.

There can be problems with the sensitivity of the NHP as a survey instrument because of the zero modal response which means that the NHP does not discriminate for a substantial proportion of the adult population. The problem with using the NHP within a population survey is that the sample would include a large number of relatively fit members who would gain low NHP scores. As it is a severe measure, minor illnesses are not detected by the instrument, and therefore minor improvements over time are unlikely to be detected. This problem was acknowledged by its authors:

The NHP is clearly tapping only the extreme end of perceived health problems. Such a distribution was built into the NHP during its development. At an early stage it was decided that it would be undesirable to include health problems which would be affirmed by a large proportion of the population.

(Hunt *et al.* 1986)

Hunt (1988) reported the proportion of zero scorers from combined data from several community studies using the NHP:

Section	Proportion of zero scores
Pain	83
Social isolation	82
Physical mobility	78
Energy	75
Emotional reactions	61
Sleep	56

As she admits, this instrument only taps the more extreme end of a distribution.

Kind and Carr-Hill (1987) used the NHP with 1,598 people in a follow-up study of the Rowntree Poverty Survey in York. The sample was weighted towards older and retired adults. Negative responses to all categories of the NHP exceeded 60 per cent, and for social isolation the figure rose to 89 per cent. Three items in particular only received 2 per cent endorsement: 'I find it hard to dress myself', 'I'm unable to walk at all', and 'I feel that life is not worth living'. Also, three of the most often cited items are drawn from the sleep category and three of the least frequently cited items are from the physical-mobility category. The authors argue that the skewness of the distribution of responses does not appear to be based on any logic. For example, nearly half of those who made just one positive response selected 'I'm waking up early in the morning', 17.5 per cent also chose 'I lose my temper easily' but no other item is chosen by more than 5 per cent of this group. In contrast, among those who scored heavily (11 or more positive responses), six items were more popular than 'I lose my temper easily'. They reported no simple relationship between the overall score and the probability of responding to any one item and that there appeared to be considerable redundancy among items.

Validity

The NHP has been tested for face, content and criterion validity and has been reported to be a satisfactory measure of subjective health status in physical, social and emotional spheres. The face and content validity of the subjective items were established on the basis of the method for devising the scale: the items were drawn from lay experiences and respondents were able to relate to them and understand the relevance of the items (Hunt et al. 1986).

There have been numerous applications of the NHP in clinical and community settings. It has been used successfully as an outcome measure with patients undergoing heart transplants in the UK (O'Brien 1988; O'Brien et al. 1988) and was found to correlate well with clinical judgements of morbidity and prognosis as well as being simple to administer and analyse.

Jenkinson et al. (1988) used both the NHP and Goldberg's General Health Questionnaire on a population of 39 rheumatoid arthritis and 43 migraine patients and reported a correlation of 0.49 between the GHQ and the emotional-reactions scale of the NHP for both samples. The implication is that the NHP is providing no more than a moderately accurate measure in this domain.

Testing for discriminative ability took place with four groups of people aged 65+; 40 people participating in a research exercise programme; 19 patients from a general practitioner (GP's) list who had no known disability or illness and who had not contacted a doctor within the prior two months; 49 people with a variety of health and social problems attending a local authority-run luncheon club; 54 chronically ill patients on GPs' lists; 352 randomly selected patients from GPs' lists. Results showed that the NHP was able to discriminate between groups of 'well' and 'ill' people, and in terms of physiological fitness; high and low GP consulters; social classes, age groups and sexes and that the content of the questions was understood by, and acceptable to, elderly people. Perceived health status was also associated with objective health status (Hunt et al. 1980; 1986).

Jenkinson et al. (1988) assessed the sensitivity of the NHP with 39 rheumatoid arthritis sufferers and 43 migraine sufferers. The NHP was able to distinguish between the two patient groups: the arthritis patients scored worse in relation to effects on energy levels and mobility. Discriminant analysis showed that the NHP was able to discriminate between 79 per cent of arthritis and 93 per cent of migraine patients.

The NHP has been shown in other studies to be sensitive to change. One unpublished study cited by Hunt et al. (1986) was based on a sample of 80 pregnant women. The NHP was administered to the women at three stages during their pregnancy – 18, 27 and 37 weeks. The NHP was sensitive to changes during pregnancy. The NHP was also administered to 141 patients attending a fracture clinic and an equal number of control subjects. Scores were obtained soon after the fracture occurred and eight weeks later. Scores were sensitive to changes in perceived health, concomitant with the healing of the fracture (McKenna et al. 1984).

Another recent application of the NHP was reported by O'Brien et al.

(1988). The authors used the instrument to measure quality of life before and after combined lung and heart transplantation in the UK. It was again sensitive to changes and correlated well with clinical measures such as exercise capacity (correlation coefficient for the latter not given). The results indicated significant reductions in NHP scores for patients at three months after surgery; no further differences were recorded at six and twelve months postoperatively.

There has been some criticism that each section does not represent just one dimension (Kind and Carr-Hill 1987; Kind mimeo). In particular, fairly high correlations between the pain and physical-mobility categories were reported. While covariation might be expected for items within categories, covariation between items in different categories raises difficulties in interpretation of a cross-category profile.

Reliability

Two studies have focused on the reliability of the NHP, using the test-retest technique. These were based on 58 patients with osteoarthritis and 93 with peripheral vascular disease. The questionnaires were repeated with these two groups at four and eight weeks after the first administration respectively. Both demonstrated a fairly high level of reliability with correlations of between 0.71 and 0.88, with the exception of the items on home life (0.64), social life (0.59), interests and hobbies (0.44) for patients with osteoarthritis; and social life (0.61), looking after the home (0.64) and work (0.55) for patients with vascular disease (Hunt *et al.* 1981; 1986). Part II of the NHP does not obtain as good results as Part I. For example, Hunt *et al.* (1981) reported that the test-retest reliability coefficients on the osteoarthritis patients ranged between 0.77 to 0.85 for Part I in comparison with a wider range for Part II at 0.44 to 0.86. The authors note that any changes in perceived health between the two administrations will consequently reduce the correlations. (Hunt *et al.* 1981). The NHP does not meet the requirements for carrying out split-half reliability as it is too short and the items are not homogeneous. The authors also argue that it is not possible to test it against an acceptable gold standard as no suitable measure exists.

A study of its adaptation into French by Bucquet *et al.* (1990) confirmed the immediate intelligibility of the French version, although it was not without problems. The authors used the same methods of calculating item weights as McKenna *et al.* (1981) for the original version, based on Thurstone's paired comparisons; their study was based on a quota sample of 625 people ('judges'). However, Bucquet *et al.* did report that the respondents had difficulties making these ratings, especially in relation to the pain, mobility, energy and sleep sections. They did not all easily grasp the concept of a 'general view' when comparing the health statements.

In sum, the advantages of the NHP are that it is short, simple and inexpensive to administer, it can be self-administered or interview based, it has been well tested for validity; partly tested for reliability and it is sensitive to change. However, it provides only a limited measure of function, and some disabilities are not assessed at all: e.g. sensory defects, incontinence, eating problems. It also lacks an adequate index of mental distress and requires supplementation if used as a broader measure of health-related quality of life. It is too short to test for split-half reliability, and it is a severe measure with a highly skewed distribution – it may not measure minor improvements in health. The result of the focus on severe conditions is that some people who are in distress may not show scores on the profile. Similarly, normally healthy persons or those with few ailments may affirm only a small number of statements on some sections. This makes it difficult to compare their scores over time. People who score zero cannot be shown to improve over time. It is a negative measure of health.

The McMaster Health Index Questionnaire (MHIQ)

The McMaster Health Index Questionnaire was developed in Ontario, Canada, as a measure of physical, social and emotional functioning. The measure was intended to provide independent measurements of these separate areas, given the authors' recognition that two individuals with the same level of physical disability may differ widely in their social and emotional functioning (Chambers *et al.* 1976). The aim was to produce a health-status questionnaire suitable for administration to general populations that could be used to predict a health professional's clinical assessment of a person's health.

The Social Function Index section was developed after consideration of existing scales, including the Spitzer Mental Status Schedule, the Cornell Medical Index and the Katz Adjustment Scale (Brodman *et al.* 1949; Herron *et al.* 1964; Spitzer *et al.* 1964), and a range of survey instruments. Review of sociological studies of leisure and social participation produced an additional list of social function questions.

The selection criteria of items included positive as well as negative discriminators (i.e. good functioning was intended to be identified); general applicability and acceptability; low cost and quick administration; quantifiable responses.

The Health Index of the questionnaire included additional items on physical function and items relating to symptoms (respiratory symptoms) and behaviour (cigarette use). Clinical assessments of social function from 'very poor' to 'very good' were included. These items were tested initially on 70 patients in an acute medical ward and repeated after their discharge. The draft questionnaire was reported to be quick and simple to administer, acceptable to respondents and sensitive to changes in health status (values unreported). Clinical assessments were repeated by an independent physician on 54 patients. Consistency ratings resulted in a Goodman–Kruskal Index of Agreement value of 0.90.

Further testing with over 200 patients registered with a family physician reported high consistency between social functioning items (dichotomizing responses into good and poor). The sensitivity of the instrument was assessed to be good. Self-completion of the final version of the McMaster Health Index Questionnaire takes 20 minutes.

The McMaster Health Index Questionnaire has been used on a number of different patient populations, including psychiatry out-patients, diabetic patients, respiratory-disease patients, patients with myocardial infarction and patients with rheumatoid arthritis (see review by Chambers 1984).

Content

The final version contains 24 physical-function items (physical activity, mobility, self-care, communication (sight, hearing), global physical function); 25 social-function items (general well-being, work/social role performance/material welfare, family support/participation, friends' support/participation and global social function); and 25 emotional function items (self-esteem, feelings toward personal relationships, thoughts about the future, critical life events and global emotional function). The MHIQ contains only 59 items as some items cover both social and emotional functions.

All the physical function items are designed to evaluate the patient's functional level on the day the MHIQ is administered. The social-function items are explicitly concerned with a specific time period (usually the present). The agree–disagree emotional-function items are phrased in the present tense. Other emotional-function items refer to the recent past as specifically defined within the question (e.g. within the last year). None of the items ask the respondent to report changes in physical, social or emotional function.

The emphasis is on ability, rather than performance ('Can you . . . ?' rather than 'Do you . . . ?'). The aim was to elicit information on activities that could be observed at the time the MHIQ was completed. Examples of questions are:

Physical:

Today, are you physically able to take part in any sports (hockey, swimming, bowling, golf, and so forth) or exercise regularly?
1 No
2 Yes

Do you have any physical difficulty at all driving a car by yourself?
1 No
2 Yes   Is this because of a physical difficulty?
  1 No
  2 Yes

Emotional health:

(strongly agree 1 _____ strongly disagree 5)

I sometimes feel that my life is not very useful.
People feel affectionate towards me.

Social health:

(good 1 _____ poor 5)

How would you say your social functioning is today? (By this we mean your ability to work, to have friends, and to get along with your family.)

How much time, in a one-week period do you usually spend watching television? (none _____ more than 2 hours a day).

Scoring

A score of 1 is given to 'good function' responses for each item, and 0 is assigned to 'poor functioning' responses. The scores are summed, although alternative weighting schemes have been developed (Chambers *et al.* 1982).

Validity

The authors reported, without publishing the values, that the MHIQ correlated well with other scales: the physical-function item correlated well with rheumatologists' and occupational therapists' assessments based on the Lee Index of Functional Capacity; the MHIQ index of emotional, physical and social function correlated well with the Bradburn Psychological Well-Being scales. The physical-function index also correlated with analogue pain scales and with clinical and biological results (Chambers *et al.* 1982).

Assessments with a group of 96 physiotherapy patients showed a change in MHIQ scores between first visit and discharge, indicating sensitivity to change (Chambers *et al.* 1982) (numbers and values unreported). A subset of the items has been successfully used to predict patient outcome in a randomized controlled trial of patients treated by nurse practitioners and doctors (Sackett *et al.* 1974).

Self-completion has been reported to be superior in terms of sensitivity to change than the other methods (Chambers *et al.* 1987). In addition, 96 patients in a physiotherapy clinic were administered the MHIQ at four points in time. Patients were randomly assigned to different modes of administration: interviewer administered, self-completion, or telephone interview. Self-completion was superior in terms of sensitivity to change than the other methods (Chambers 1984).

Reliability

Chambers (1984) reported that reliability was assessed by asking 30 physiotherapy out-patients to complete the MHIQ on two occasions within a one-week period. Patients were not expected to change in their functional status. The correlation between the physical and emotional function values was 0.80. Intraclass correlation coefficients ranged from 0.48 to 0.95 for the physical, emotional and social scores. Internal consistency coefficients between the physical, emotional and social functional indices were 0.76, 0.67 and 0.51 respectively. Reliability was not affected by self- or interviewer-administered scales.

In sum, the advantages of the scale are its flexibility – it can be used in different settings; it is amenable to mathematical scoring contruction; it focuses on present ability; it is positive in orientation; it is simple and inexpensive to administer, and acceptable to patients. It also has an acceptable level of reliability. However, it is of questionable applicability to the very elderly (e.g. question on sports participation in physical index). More studies of its reliability and validity are also needed.

THE RAND HEALTH INSURANCE STUDY BATTERIES

The Rand Corporation's health batteries were designed for the Rand Health Insurance Study (HIS), an experiment of health outcome following random allocation to various insurance plans among adults aged 14–61 years. The batteries were developed for use in population surveys. More specifically, the Rand Health Insurance Study batteries were developed as an outcome measure to detect changes in health status that might be expected to occur as a result of health-service use within a relatively short period of time. The batteries cover physical health, physiological health mental health, social health and perceptions of health. The measures were intended to be sensitive to differences in health in general populations (Ware and Karmos 1976; Stewart et al. 1978; 1981; 1989; Ware et al. 1979; 1980).

The HIS is based on a sample of about 8,000 people in 2,750 families in six sites across the USA. The HIS batteries were developed after extensive reserch into existing measures and testing of adaptations of existing measures or of new measures developed on the basis of extensive reviews of the literature. Each section can be used independently. Their use has been largely confined to populations in the USA. The scale has not yet been tested on elderly people.

Apart from the ongoing Rand Health Insurance Study, there have been few other applications of the Rand batteries. One of these few applications was carried out in two general practices in Sydney, Australia, by Hall *et al.* (1987). The Rand instruments were tested against the Sickness Impact Profile (SIP) and the General Health Questionnaire (GHQ). All instruments were reported to be acceptable to patients and the refusal rate was low.

Remaining applications are confined to the Rand studies. The authors have a wide range of publicly available reports of findings to date, and some published papers which show the interrelationships between the HIS batteries (Stewart *et al.* 1989; Wells *et al.* 1989). A short 20-item version of the batteries has been developed (Stewart *et al.* 1988), although this has now been overtaken by a 36-item version (the Short-Form 36), which is attracting international interest and is also being piloted in the UK (Anderson *et al.* 1990; Stewart and Ware (in press).

Physical Health Battery

In the Health Insurance Study physical health was operationalized in terms of functional status. A review of the literature revealed six categories of functional activity for which performance has been assumed to reflect physical health: self-care (e.g. feeding, bathing), mobility, physical activities, role activities (e.g. employment), household activities and leisure activities. These six areas were thus incorporated into the Rand battery, called the Functional Limitations Battery. These items in the Functional Limitations Battery were based on items from the US National Health Interview Survey and Patrick *et al.*'s (1973a; 1973b) work on developing functional ability scales. Performance was measured by three separate batteries of items: functional limitations, physical abilities and disability days.

An advantage of the Rand Functional Limitations Battery over other scales is that it relates the scale to the cause of the physical incapacity, that is where patients are aware of diagnostic causes.

The Rand Physical Health Battery includes the Physical Abilities Battery in addition to the Functional Limitations Battery. These are similar to each other and were intended to be administered to respondents at different stages of the longitudinal HIS.

Content

Fourteen HIS items assess activities in self-care, mobility, physical, household and leisure activities, and role activities.

Response choices are either 'yes' or 'no' or 'yes, can do', 'yes, can do but only slowly', 'no, unable to do'. Positive responses to problems lead to further items on length of restriction.

Examples from the (revised) Functional Limitations Battery and Physical Abilities Battery are:

Does your health limit the kind of vigorous activities you can do, such as running, lifting heavy objects, or participating in strenuous sports?   Yes   1/No   2

Do you have any trouble either walking several blocks or climbing a few flights of stairs, because of your health?   Yes   1/No   2

Do you need help with eating, dressing, bathing, or using the toilet because of your health?   Yes   1/No   2

Can you do hard activities at home, heavy work like scrubbing floors, or lifting or moving heavy furniture?   Yes   1/Yes, but only slowly   2/No, I can't do this   3

If you wanted to, could you participate in active sports such as swimming, tennis, basketball, volleyball, or rowing a boat?   Yes   1/Yes, but only slowly   2/No, I can't do this   3.

Many of these items are inapplicable to very elderly people (e.g. strenuous sports activity) or are too general (e.g. asking about several limitations in the same question) to be useful in surveys where discriminative ability is important.

Scoring

Item score ranges vary: 0–3 (none to more severe limitations) for mobility; 0–4 for physical limitations; 0–2 for role limitations. Items can be scored in groups: mobility limitations, role limitations, self-care limitations (the latter included only one item). An overall score – the Functional Status Index – utilizes all items and is an index of the number of categories in which a person has one or more limitations (0–4). This has not been fully tested for validity.

Results from the Rand study showed that the physical health measures yielded skewed distributions: most sample members had no functional limitations or physical disabilities. This is a limitation regarding its suitability for use in population surveys.

Validity

The authors judged the measure to have acceptable content validity as the content of items included in the physical-health measures reflected the range of content reported in the literature. Construct validity was assumed by the authors as associations between the Functional Limitations Battery and the Physical Abilities Battery were moderate to strong (0.49–0.99), indicating an underlying general construct, presumably physical health.

Reliability

Reliability was estimated for the physical-abilities measures using internal-consistency coefficients. The internal-consistency and reproducibility coefficients for HIS measures of physical health were high (0.90 or above); test-retest coefficients (at four months apart) were also high (0.92–0.99).

Mental Health Battery

As a result of an extensive literature review, ranging from assessments of depression scales to general well-being schedules, the measurement of symptoms of affective (mood) disorders (e.g. depression, anxiety) was considered important, as well as well-being and self-control of behaviour, moods, thought and feelings. The HIS Mental Health Battery contains items hypothesized to measure these constructs. It has been revised since its development in order to extend the range of measurement (particularly with anxiety and depression).

Content

The Revised Mental Health Battery is constructed from the General Well-Being Questionnaire. A new sub-scale has been added defining loss of behavioural/emotional control. The revised version was based on factor analyses. The General Well-Being Questionnaire comprises 46 questions with four to six response choices for each item, ranging from extremely positive to extremely negative evaluations. The Mental Health Battery utilizes 38 of these questions; the remaining eight items are used to estimate socially desirable responses. Examples of items are:

How much have you been bothered by nervousness or your 'nerves' during the past month?

Extremely so – to the point where I could not work or take care of things	1
Very much bothered	2
Bothered quite a bit by nerves	3
Bothered some – enough to bother me	4
Bothered just a little by nerves	5
Not bothered at all by this	6

During the past month, have you had any reason to wonder if you were losing your mind, or losing control over the way you act, talk, think, feel, or of your memory?

No, not at all   1
Maybe a little   2
Yes, but not enough to be concerned or worried about it 3
Yes, and I have been a little concerned   4
Yes, and I am quite concerned   5
Yes, and I am very much concerned about it   6

In general, would you say your morals have been above reproach?

Yes, definitely   1
Yes, probably   2
I don't know   3
Probably not   4
Definitely not   5

How often have you felt like crying, during the past month?

Always   1
Very often   2
Fairly often   3
Sometimes   4
Almost never   5
Never   6

Scoring

Eight items measure social desirability and should be scored separately from the 38 Mental Health Index items.

Some items are recoded for scoring purposes. Sub-scales can be created relating to a life-satisfaction item; a psychological-distress scale; a psychological well-being scale and the mental-health index. This involves the simple addition of item scores and the recoded scores. High scores are interpreted differently for different sub-scales, according to the scale name; for example, a high score for a negative scale corresponds with an unfavourable score and a high score for a positive scale corresponds with a favourable score. Full details of the scoring method are available from the authors at Rand Corporation, Santa Monica.

Validity

The content validity of the HIS Mental Health Battery was assumed by the authors as it contained items represented in the literature. Construct validity is more questionable as correlations between these scales and those constructed for validity studies ranged from 0–0.01 to 0.94. This reflects doubt about the measurement of a common construct within the scale. The authors use these findings to support their decision to score and interpret separately the four construct specific mental-health scales. An Australian community survey by Hall *et al.* (1987) reported a correlation of –0.76 between the Rand Mental Health Battery and the General Health Questionnaire which largely assesses depression and anxiety.

Reliability

The reliability of the HIS mental-health measures was estimated using internal-consistency and test-retest coefficients. Internal consistency estimates were fairly high (0.72–0.94). Test-retest estimates ranged from 0.70 to 0.80, the time period between administrations being generally less than one week. A more recent development is a brief 8-item depression scale, with initially promising results for reliability and validity (Burnam *et al.* 1988; Wells *et al.* 1989).

The Social Health Battery

The Social Health Battery was developed alongside the other Rand health measures assessing physical and psychological status.

On the basis of the literature again, social health was operationally defined in terms of interpersonal interactions. The Social Health Battery measures social well-being and support, operationalized by measuring social interaction and resources. The two main dimensions of the eleven-item battery are the number of social resources a person has, and the frequency with which s/he has contact with relatives and friends.

Content

The scale covers home, family, friendships, social and community life. It does not cover satisfaction with relationships. The scale has been described by Donald and Ware (1982). Questions include:

About how many close friends do you have – people you feel at ease with and can talk with about what is on your mind? (You may include relatives.)

During the past month, about how often have you had friends over to your home? (Do not count relatives.)

Every day.
Several days a week.
About once a week.
Two or three times in the past month.
Once in the past month.
Not at all in the past month.

And how often were you on the telephone with close friends or relatives during the past month?

Every day.
Several times a week.
About once a week.
Two or three times.
Once.
Not at all.

An additional item asks about frequency of letter writing but the authors advise dropping this item as so few people answer in the affirmative at all.

Scoring

An overall social support score utilizes all the items (except letter writing and a general question asking about how the person gets on with others). This scoring has not been fully tested for validity.

Validity

Data about validity was drawn from 4,603 interviews from the Health Insurance Study. The Social Health Battery is judged by its authors to have content validity in so far as it reflects the two major components of social health identified in the literature: interpersonal interaction and social participation. The authors do not attempt to include any of the other areas of social health; thus content validity is only partial.

Criterion validity was tested by using the items in the scale and a nine-item self-rating of health, a measure of emotional ties and a nine-item psychological-well-being scale. The correlations were low. Further evidence of the validity of the battery is required.

Reliability

The inter-item correlations arc low. Test-retest coefficients are moderate and range from 0.55 to 0.68. Further testing for reliability is required.

The results for reliability and validity are not so far convincing. Further testing is required. The large-scale and longitudinal nature of the Rand HIS study offers exciting possibilities for further testing and development of the measure.

General Health Perceptions Battery

This asks respondents for an assessment or self-rating of their health in general (Stewart *et al.* 1978; Davies and Ware 1981). These are defined in the HIS with respect to time (perceptions of prior, current and future health) and with respect to three other constructs indicative of general health perceptions, including resistance or susceptibility to illness, health worry and concern, and sickness orientation (the extent to which people perceive illness to be a part of their lives).

A major strength of the General Health Perceptions Battery is ease of administration. Self-administration of this section takes approximately seven minutes. It is of potential use in studies attempting to predict the use of medical services.

Content

The battery contains 29 items, 26 of which were taken from the Health Perceptions Questionnaire developed by Ware and Karmos (1976) for the National Center for Health Services Research.

The items include statements of opinion about personal health (e.g. 'I expect to have a very healthy life'), accompanied by five standardized response categories defining a true–false continuum: definitely true, mostly true, don't know, mostly false, definitely false. These items are used to score six sub-scales assessing different dimensions of health perceptions: past health, present health, future health, health-related worries and concerns, resistance or susceptibility to illness and the tendency to view illness as part of life. Examples of items are:

I try to avoid letting illness interfere with my life.
I will probably be sick a lot in the future.
I don't like going to the doctor.
I'm not as healthy as I used to be.
When I'm sick, I try to just keep going as usual.
I expect to have a very healthy life.
When I think I am getting sick, I fight it.

It is apparent from these questions that analyses need to control for age, especially in relation to expectations about the future and current health status.

Scoring

All items are scored to produce a global figure, although the scoring has not been fully tested for validity. Distributions appear to be fairly normal. Hall *et al.* (1987) reported the Rand measures to be less skewed than the SIP or GHQ.

Validity

The measure of health perceptions was reported by the authors to be correlated with the physical, mental and social health batteries (coefficients unreported). In the Australian study by Hall *et al*. (1987) the Rand batteries relating to general health perceptions were tested on 160 patients along with the Sickness Impact Profile and the General Health Questionnaire. A correlation of −0.30 was considered to be the threshold for assessment of relationships between the three instruments. The Rand mental-health index was reported to correlate weakly to moderately well with three of the SIP components (emotional behaviour): −0.32 to −0.54. To some extent the same constructs are being measured, although these correlations are not high. If 0.50 is taken as the minimum correlation coefficient for validity acceptance for group studies, then the instruments tested do not achieve this (Ware *et al*. 1980). On the other hand, it was reported previously that the GHQ correlated highly with the Rand Mental Health Battery (−0.76) (Hall *et al*. 1987).

The stability of the Health Perceptions Battery has been estimated for intervals of one, two and three years between administrations. The median stability coefficients for one, two and three years for adults are 0.66, 0.59 and 0.56 respectively. Further tests are ongoing for reliability and validity. Preliminary results suggest that it can discriminate between those with and without a chronic disease, is sensitive to individual differences in disease severity, and is sensitive to changes over time in both physical and mental functioning.

Hall *et al*. (1987) reported that of the three instruments used in the Australian study (the Rand instrument, the SIP and the GHQ), the Rand measures had the best discriminative ability and were reported by the authors to be preferred as a general health status measure in a general population.

Reliability

The reliability of the Health Perceptions Questionnaire scale was estimated using internal consistency and test-retest coefficients. These were tested by its authors using a non-HIS population. Test-retest reliability estimates were based on data collected approximately six weeks apart from the same respondents. Results indicate that the scale was more reliable than single-item measures, although internal-consistency co-efficients (unreported) were lower than for test-retest. Internal consistency for the scale generally exceeded 0.50 (sometimes 0.90). More extensive testing of the Rand instruments is still required.

The Cornell Medical Index (CMI)

The Cornell Medical Index was initially designed for use by physicians in medical-history taking in order to save their time and ensure, where appropriate, that a large body of medical and psychiatric data could be collected. It was intended to serve as a standardized medical history (Brodman *et al.* 1949). The informal language used on the instrument was intended to be readily translatable into medical terminology. For example: 'Does your heart often race like mad?' (tachycardia); 'Do you have to get up every night and urinate (pass water)?' (nocturia).

In the process of its development, many variations of the CMI items were tested on more than a thousand people in several geographic areas. Those items containing replies substantiated on interview were included in the final version. The final form was tested on 179 medical out-patients and 191 admitted medical patients whose responses were compared with their medical histories taken by participating physicians. Although the index was intended for use as an aid to medical-history taking in clinic and hospital settings, the authors state that it could also be useful in population-health surveys.

One published study of the CMI, based on 5,119 patients reported that, as would be expected, older people reported more physical problems than younger people; and that women reported more problems than men, although they had a similar number of diagnosed disorders (Brodman *et al.* 1953). There are numerous examples of the application of the CMI in clinic and institutional settings. Comprehensive references on applications of the index have been compiled by Cornell Medical University and are available on request (Lowe 1975). Abramson *et al.* (1965) summarized the CMI scores reported for 16 samples of people studied in the USA and UK. Reported CMI scores of 30+ ranged between 4 and 82 per cent for female sample members, and between 0 and 79 per cent for males. The populations studied ranged widely from psychiatric hospital out-patients to people labelled as 'healthy'.

The CMI is self-administered. Individuals usually take 10 to 30 minutes to complete it. The authors report that the time taken to complete the CMI depends on people's level of education, and the speed at which they reach decisions. They report the CMI to be acceptable to patients. No training is needed for administration or analysis.

Content

The CMI contains 195 yes–no questions divided into 18 sections relating to physical problems (8 sections), personal habits, frequency of illness (4 sections), moods and feelings (6 sections).

The sections of the CMI are:

A Eyes and ears
B Respiratory system
C Cardiovascular system

D Digestive tract
E Musculoskeletal system
F Skin
G Nervous system
H Genito-urinary system
I   Fatigability
J   Frequency of illness
K Miscellaneous disease
L Habits

Mood and feelings:

M Inadequacy
N Depression
O Anxiety
P Sensitivity
Q Anger
R Tension

Examples of questions are:

Does your face often get badly flushed?   Yes/No
Do you suffer badly from frequent severe headaches?   Yes/No
Do you usually feel bloated after eating?   Yes/No
Has a doctor ever said you have kidney or bladder disease?   Yes/No
Did anyone in your family ever have a nervous breakdown?   Yes/No
Do you often feel unhappy and depressed?   Yes/No

There are two forms of the CMI, one for men and one for women (differing only in the genito-urinary section). The number of problems admitted are scored and the total number indicates the degree of deviancy.

Scoring

Responses indicating the existence of a problem (the 'yes' replies) are totalled. More than 25 positive responses to items indicate the presence of serious disorder. A medically significant emotional disturbance is considered present if the total score is 30 or more. If the 'yes' replies are chiefly located in one or two sections, the medical problem is localized. If they are scattered throughout the index, the problem is likely to be diffused, usually involving a medical disturbance. More than two or three 'yes' answers on the last page (moods, feelings, attitudes and behaviour questions) suggest a psychological disturbance. However, interpretation of symptoms depends on medical knowledge and thus the index is not a useful diagnostic tool outside medical settings.

Validity and reliability

Although this is an extremely popular measure, there are few reports of the instrument's reliability and validity. Abramson *et al.* (1965) point out that the index is of little value in comparisons of widely divergent cultures within and between societies.

Brodman   *et al.* (1954), in a study of 7,527 men undergoing medical examination, including the administration of the CMI, for army training, analysed the follow-up records of 900 of them four months later, after their commencement of training. High CMI scores (50+) were significantly associated with a large amount of reported sickness, hospitalized days, convictions and discharges from the service.

A study of its validity was undertaken by Abramson *et al.* (1965) among 120 randomly selected adults of a Jerusalem housing project. The authors tested its sensitivity and specificity, the former in relation to the proportion of unhealthy persons who gave the defined CMI response ('yes' to items), and specificity in terms of the proportion of healthy persons who did not give this response. Health status was independently assessed by local physicians. The authors reported that the responses to individual CMI questions referring to named disorders were not very valid indicators of the presence of these disorders. Of the people whom physicians reported as having a specific condition, only a half, or in some cases less than a half, of these people themselves reported its presence. The conditions were, on the other hand, rarely reported by people who were assessed by physicians as not having them. Although item responses were not judged to be valid indicators, scores (based on the number of 'yes' responses) were significantly correlated with the physicians' ratings of overall ill health and emotional ill health, although the correlations were weak to moderate (0.26 – 0.48). Moderate correlations were also obtained between physicians' ratings of emotional and overall health (0.52 for women and 0.57 for men); 78 per cent of the people rated as 'ill' by physicians were also rated by them as emotionally disturbed. In addition, the authors identified the ten key questions which were the best predictors of physician ratings of emotional ill health; there was a moderate correlation between the number of these items with positive scores and total CMI scores (0.63):

Are you easily upset and irritated?
Do you suffer from severe nervous exhaustion?
Do you usually have great difficulty in falling asleep or staying asleep?
Are you definitely underweight?
Do you often become suddenly scared for no good reason?
Are you considered a nervous person?
Are you constantly keyed up and jittery?
Do you usually feel unhappy and depressed?

Does life look entirely hopeless?
Does every little thing get on your nerves and wear you out?

The general findings of the study that the CMI is of limited value for the detection of specific disorders was also confirmed by a large-scale study in New York by Brodman et al. (1959). They compared the results of medical examinations of 5,929 hospital out-patients with computer analyses of the CMI for the same patients. These authors reported that CMI data provided correct diagnoses of 60 common disorders in only 44 per cent of cases known to have these disorders.

The instrument needs further testing if it is to be used in survey research, although evidence of the validity of individual items is not encouraging; it is also fairly limited in so far as it concentrates mainly on symptom reporting regarding mental and physical problems, rather than perceptions of health and well-being.

Spitzer's Quality of Life Index (QL)

Spitzer's Quality of Life Index was developed for use by physicians in relation to cancer and chronically ill patients and is widely used by cancer specialists interested in the health status and quality of life of their patients before and after therapy.

Spitzer et al. (1981) aimed to identify the components of quality of life empirically from questioning lay people as well as health professionals. They formed three advisory panels each with 43 members from Sydney, Australia. These consisted of cancer patients and their relatives, patients with chronic diseases and their relatives, healthy people aged between 20–59 and 60+, physicians, nurses, social workers and other health professionals and members of the clergy. One panel received an open-ended questionnaire designed to elicit spontaneous beliefs about factors that could enhance or decrease the quality of life. The second panel received a more structured questionnaire seeking views on various aspects of defined quality of life. The third panel assessed the results from the first two and the relative importance of the main factors. The factors that were rated as the most important formed the first drafts of the QL Index which were tested on 339 subjects from out-patients' clinics. This resulted in the following dimensions of quality of life being incorporated within the definitive QL Index: activity; performance of activities of daily living; perception of health; support from family and friends; and outlook on life.

Its authors caution that it is not suitable for measuring or classifying the quality of life of ostensibly healthy people (Spitzer et al. 1981). The average completion time is one minute.

Content

The QL consists of five items. Each item represents a different domain of life functioning from which the respondents choose in terms of the statement's applicability to themselves: activity, daily living, health, support and outlook. These were agreed by a panel of experts to be crucial areas of life functioning. The index is short and easily administered.

The scale also comprises a visual-analogue rating scale and requests the respondent and interviewer to place an X on the line rating quality of life (lowest quality–highest quality).

Respondents are requested to tick statements which apply to them. There are many examples of multiple items within one question and thus this scale confuses several activities within one item:

I am able to eat, wash, go to the toilet and dress without assistance. I drive a car or use public transport without assistance.

I work full time (or nearly so) in my usual occupation or study full-time (or nearly so) or manage my own household or take part in as much unpaid or voluntary activity as I wish, whether retired or not.

I have good relationships with others and receive strong support from at least one family member and/or friend.

I am basically a calm person. I generally look forward to things and am able to make my own decisions about my life and surroundings.

Respondents only have the option of one tick per statement to indicate they can do all of these things, or of not ticking to indicate they cannot do any without assistance. There are problems with interpretation if respondents can do some tasks but not others.

Scoring

The scoring of the Spitzer QL scale is simple. The scale consists of five items, with three options for replies. The item responses comprise scores 0–2, giving an overall score of 0 to 10. The scale can be summed into a single score or each item can be presented separately.

Validity

Spitzer et al. (1981) asked 68 lay people and professionals (e.g. physicians) to assess the scope and format of the instrument; most judged it to be satisfactory and the authors judged the scale to have content validity.

Spitzer et al. (1981) tested the scale for validity, using 150 physicians to rate 879 patients. Fifty-nine per cent of physicians reported that they were 'very confident' of the accuracy of their scores. The analysis of physicians' scores showed that the close clustering of high scores among healthy subjects, the spread of scores among those who were definitely ill, and the low scores of those who were seriously ill, made clinical sense and provided evidence of discriminant construct validity. Convergent validity was judged to be obtained by comparison of physicians' and patients' ratings. When the physicians' ratings were compared to patients' self-ratings, the correlation was moderately high (0.61). The scale is also related to other global-functioning scales (Mor *et al.* 1984; Morris *et al.* 1986; Mor 1987). Mor (1987), on the basis of three samples of newly diagnosed cancer patients (total: 2,046), reported a correlation between the Spitzer QL Index and the Karnofsky Performance Scale of 0.63; the correlation was moderate probably because of the multidimensional nature of the QL Index. The item correlations of the scale with the Karnofsky Scale ranged from 0.13 to 0.57. The scale and the associated visual-analogue scale has been primarily evaluated in two other main studies which showed a statistically significant correlation with other indices (Spitzer *et al.* 1981; Gough *et al.* 1983). However, the correlation coefficients were not high enough to be confident that these scales cover the same dimensions. The scale's reproducibility requires further investigation. The authors reported that the scale was able to discriminate between healthy people and patients with varying conditions.

However, Slevin *et al.* (1988) concluded on the basis of their analyses that the doctors' ratings of quality of life using the Spitzer scale were of questionable validity. They reported that the Spitzer scale contained inappropriate questions for measuring the quality of life of cancer patients. They suggest that the continued popularity of the Spitzer scale, despite poor reliability and validity of the scales, stems from researchers' tendency to rely on significance values when assessing their scales, rather than on the size of the correlation value.

The Spitzer scale has been reported to be able to predict mortality among cancer patients (Mor *et al.* 1984; Morris *et al.* 1986; Mor 1987). It has been used in an Australian study of outcome of breast-cancer patients and was shown to be capable of discriminating between patients on intermittent therapy and those receiving continuous therapy (Coates *et al.* 1987).

There are numerous applications of this scale in clinical settings. Morris and Sherwood (1987) in the USA administered the QL scale to different samples of cancer patients at different stages of the disease. Over 2,000 patients were included in the study. A strong correlation was reported between the Karnofsky performance-status rating and the QL Index. The QL Index was able to successfully distinguish between cancer patients who were newly diagnosed, those under active treatment and those nearing the terminal stages of the disease. However, the authors did not feel it was sufficiently sensitive for use as an outcome variable in studies evaluating the effect of a treatment or intervention on patients' lives. This was mainly because of the insensitivity of the social-functioning index of the scale.

The QL's reliance on just five items means that it does not adequately account for the different dimensions of quality of life. However, to be fair, the authors did not intend it to be appropriate for measuring global quality of life in healthy populations, and they reported that it does not discriminate adequately among well people (Spitzer *et al.* 1981).

Reliability

Spitzer *et al.* (1981), on the basis of 150 physicians' ratings of 879 patients, reported that assessment of internal consistency demonstrated a high coefficient (0.77), and the correlation for inter-rater reliability was high (0.81). The scale has been shown to have reasonable inter-item reliability (Mor *et al.* 1984; Morris *et al.* 1986; Mor 1987).

However, there are few other studies of its reliability and validity. Slevin *et al.* (1988) administered the index along with the Linear Analogue Self-Assessment (LASA) quality-of-life visual-analogue scales, the Karnofsky Performance Scale, and the Hospital Anxiety and Depression Scale. The scales were completed by 108 patients and their doctors at the same time. Two different groups of 25 patients filled in the same questionnaires on a single day, and daily for five consecutive days. Reproducibility was not as good as the Karnofsky Scale. The Karnofsky Scale, which correlated with the Spitzer Index (patients' rating of quality of life: 0.49), demonstrated greater reproducibility than any of the other scales. The variability in their results from repeated testing calls into question the reliability of the Spitzer QL Index and the other measures administered.

In sum, the initial testing of the scale appeared to show promising results; the scale is able to predict mortality among cancer patients and is related to other global-functioning scales. However, more recent studies of the scale report that it has questionable reliability, and validity (Slevin *et al.* 1988). Further testing is required; a major disadvantage is the confusion of several dimensions within one item.

Linear Analogue Self Assessment (LASA)

The Linear Analogue Self Assessment Scale was developed for use with cancer patients and has been used successfully to evaluate quality of life of patients receiving cytotoxic therapy for advanced breast cancer (Priestman and Baum 1976). Although simple, it is apparently lengthy in terms of administration time.

Content

The LASA questionnaire has 25 items, 10 of which relate to the symptoms and effects of the disease and treatment (e.g. pain and nausea); 5 examine psychological consequences (e.g. anxiety and depression); 5 measure other physical indices (e.g. ability to perform household chores); and 5 items are concerned with personal relationships.

The LASA tests employ lines, the length of which are taken to denote the continuum of some emotional or physical experience such as tiredness or anxiety (Priestman and Baum 1976). The lines are usually 10 cm long with stops at right angles to the line at its extremes, representing the limits of the experience being measured. It is a technique that has been easily administered to 5-year-old children (Scott *et al.* 1977). Examples of items are:

Ability to perform shopping:
None L⎯⎯⎯⎦Better than ever

Decision making:
ImpossibleL⎯⎯⎯⎦Excellent

Nausea:
Constant L⎯⎯⎯⎦None

Appetite:
None L⎯⎯⎯⎦Excellent

How would you rate your quality of life?:
Very poorL⎯⎯⎯⎦Very good

Scoring

The patient is instructed to mark along the line a point that corresponds to his/her perception of the experience. The distance from the 'none at all' mark to the patient's mark provides a numeric score for the item. The items are summed.

Validity

There are many references in the literature to the validity of LASA in the measurement of pain (Melzack 1983). Slevin *et al.* (1988) in their testing of the scale, however, reported that the LASA scale correlated poorly with the Hospital Anxiety and Depression (HAD) scale. Slevin *et al.* suggested that this was due to the HAD items being less applicable to cancer patients.

The scale has been shown to be capable of discriminating between breast-cancer patients in Australia who receive intermittent therapy and those receiving continuous therapy (Coates *et al.* 1987).

Gough *et al.* (1983) assessed 100 patients with advanced cancer in Australia, using a single LASA item 'How would you rate your general feeling of well-being today?', a 21-item version of the LASA index, self- and interviewer-administered 5-item QL Index (Spitzer's) which covered activity, daily living, health, support and outlook. Each patient was evaluated four times at four-weekly intervals for twelve weeks. The correlation coefficients for the four methods ranged from 0.38 to 0.86. The single item LASA question correlated moderately to well with all three questionnaires (0.38 to 0.67). The LASA-21 correlated from 0.46 to –0.65 with the other items.

Reliability

The test-retest correlations of the LASA were 0.73 (Priestman and Baum 1976). Slevin *et al.* (1988) tested LASA against the Hospital Anxiety and Depression scale, the Karnofsky Index and the Spitzer Quality of Life Index with 108 cancer patients in London and reported that the LASA scale showed similar concordance coefficients when taken as a whole, compared with being divided into four equal parts, i.e. the continuous scale is no more sensitive than the four-point scale. Two different groups of 25 patients also filled in the same forms on a single day, and daily for five consecutive days, during a period when their clinical state was expected to remain stable. Professionals also completed the scales in relation to the same patients. The LASA scale was found to be easily reproducible, and had greater reproducibility than the other scales. Little other information about its reliability has been published.

Although the scale is simple and reported to be reproducible and able to discriminate between groups, it may be problematic to administer because some patients may take some time to accustom themselves to representing their feelings along a continuum. More evidence of its validity is required.

The McGill Pain Questionnaire (MPQ)

Many health-status and disability measures fail to incorporate a comprehensive assessment of pain. Apart from visual-analogue rating scales to assess pain, the most frequently used and most tested of the measures that exist to assess pain is the McGill Pain Questionnaire (MPQ). The McGill Pain Questionnaire consists principally of lists of terms describing the quality and intensity of pain. Melzack and Torgerson (1971) selected 102 words describing pain from the literature, sorted them into the categories of sensory, affective and evaluative words describing intensity; the results were then checked by 20 reviewers. Further testing among 140 students, 20 physicians and 20 patients led to the current format of the scale and the scale values. Several versions of the scale exist, and a short version of the scale has also been developed which consists of 15 items (Melzack 1987). The completion of the full-length scale takes from 5 to 15 minutes, and the short version takes 2 to 5 minutes, depending on the familiarity of the patients with the words.

Content

Examples of the words respondents are asked to choose from to describe their pain are:

Flickering
Quivering
Pulsing
Throbbing
Beating
Pounding

Tight
Numbing
Drawing
Squeezing
Tearing

The short version includes only the items throbbing, shooting, stabbing, sharp, cramping, gnawing, hot-burning, aching, heavy, tender, splitting, tiring-exhausting, sickening, fearful, punishing-cruel.

Scoring

Each description carries a weight corresponding to the severity of the pain, according to evaluations of appropriate ordinal rankings by panels of doctors, patients and students. Subjects then receive pain scores according to the number of descriptive items they select to describe their pain and their assigned weights (0=no pain; 1=mild pain; 2=discomforting; 3=distressing; 4=horrible; 5=excruciating). The McGill Pain Questionnaire generates four sub-scales differentiated by factor analysis. These include sensory and evaluative sub-scales to designate perception of pain, and an affective sub-scale to denote emotional response to pain. The scale was developed in recognition of these distinct components of pain.

There are four possible and distinct scoring methods ranging from the number of words chosen to the sum of the scale values (based on the scale weights) for all the words selected in a given category or across all categories (Melzack 1975).

Validity

Dubuisson and Melzack (1976) reported that the McGill Pain Questionnaire was able to correctly classify 77 per cent of 95 patients with eight pain syndromes into diagnostic groups on the basis of their verbal description of pain.

Correlations between McGill Pain Questionnaire score and visual-analogue ratings for 40 patients ranged from 0.50 to 0.65 (Melzack 1975). There is support from results of principal components analysis for the distinction between affective and sensory dimensions of pain, but less for a distinctive evaluative component (Prieto and Geisinger 1983; Reading 1979). The short version correlates consistently highly with the long version of the McGill Pain Questionnaire (Melzack 1987).

The specificity of the measure was demonstrated by Greenwald (1987) in a study of 536 cancer patients.

Reliability

Evidence of reliability is sparse (Graham *et al.* 1980). Melzack (1975) reported a test-retest study, based on just ten patients who completed the scale three times at intervals of three to seven days between each. The average consistency of response was reported to be 70.3 per cent.

Although it is difficult to demonstrate that the McGill Pain Questionnaire does reflect the conceptual definition of pain as three distinct dimensions, it is still the leading measure of pain.

5
Measures of psychological well-being

There are numerous scales of psychological well-being, in particular those which are aimed specifically at detecting common psychiatric disorders such as anxiety/depression, dementia and mental confusion. The reliability of the classifications of many of these have been questioned. Gold standards for diagnostic categorization have been developed over the years, for example, the revised Diagnostic and Statistical Manual (DSM-III) of the American Psychiatric Association or the International Classification of Diseases, as well as the previously developed and highly regarded Present State Examination and the Research Diagnostic Criteria (Wing *et al.* 1974; Spitzer *et al.* 1978), although these still fail to account realistically for features of personality or physical illness which may intervene. In the UK the Geriatric Mental State Questionnaire (GMS) has been developed for use with the elderly and is often regarded as a gold-standard survey instrument; the GMS is reviewed in this chapter. A more recently developed and tested assessment schedule for the diagnosis of mental disorder, although again only in relation to the elderly, is the Cambridge Examination for Mental Disorders of the Elderly (CAMDEX) (Roth *et al.* 1986). This also pays special attention to the detection of dementia. However, it is extremely long and unwieldy, and unsuitable for use as a research tool except in a clinical psychiatric survey; it compares unfavourably with other well-developed scales in relation to cross-cultural applicability and sensitivity (Copeland 1990).

The following sections review the most popular and easily administered scales of common psychiatric disorders in current use in the UK: anxiety/depression and, among the elderly, mental confusion.

Scales of psychiatric status are generally developed and applied within specific countries. It is often difficult for such scales to have cross-cultural applicability without careful adaptation because of culture specific concepts and values, although some of the more popular scales have been adapted for use outside the UK (e.g. the General Health Questionnaire and the Geriatric Mental State).

Depression

The term depression is increasingly used to cover a wider range of psychological disturbances. There is considerable confusion about the variety of meanings and this, in turn, has led to conflicting research findings about aetiology and treatment of choice (Snaith 1987). There is little confusion about the recognition of a severe state, sometimes called a psychosis, but milder degrees of the condition lack definition. Sometimes the term 'depressive neurosis' is used but a variety of concepts are associated with this term. In the Present State Examination manual, Wing et al. (1974) have provided the most succinct definitions of psychopathological terms, and in an attempt to clarify the issues of terminology their definitions of depressive states related to depressed mood, recent loss of interest, self-depreciation, hopelessness and observed depression. There were a number of additional definitions provided for neglect due to brooding, subjective anergia, slowness and underactivity, inefficient thinking, poor concentration, suicidal plans or acts, morning depression, social withdrawal, guilt and other related symptoms.

Wide discrepancies in the early literature on estimates of the prevalence of mental illness in different communities were largely the consequence of the use of different diagnostic criteria. The development and use of standardized research instruments linked to clearly stated diagnostic criteria led to less variation between studies. However, considerable differences still exist between measures with the implication that comparisons between studies can be made only if two studies have utilized the same basic measurement scale.

Many research studies have based the definition of a 'case' of depression on a certain score having been attained on one of the large number of depression-rating scales. The different construction of these scales and the different individual items they include create major difficulties in comparing studies, unless they have been developed in relation to clear criteria such as the DSM-III.

The majority of depression-rating scales contain a diverse collection of symptoms, attitudes and feelings and will produce high prevalence rates and a large proportion of false positives if case detection relies upon them (Snaith 1987). Kutner et al. (1985), studying depression and anxiety in dialysis patients, found that scales containing disease-related items yielded exaggerated scores.

Zung's Self Rating Depression Scale

The Self Rating Scale was developed by Zung (1965). It was constructed on the basis of the clinical diagnostic criteria most commonly used to characterize depressive disorders. Factor-analysis-derived symptom clusters led to the selection of 20 items covering 'pervasive affect', 'physiological equivalents or concomitants' and 'psychological concomitants'. Altogether over half of the items of this widely used depression scale are composed of feelings or symptoms which do not necessarily indicate the presence of a psychological disorder, and Kutner et al. (1985) found that these disease items led to an exaggerated score.

Content

The scale contains 20 statements; 10 are worded symptomatically positive and 10 are worded symptomatically negative. Respondents are asked how the listed statements apply to them. Administration is by self-completion; and completion time is 'a few minutes' (Zung et al. 1965). Examples are:

I have trouble sleeping at night.
I eat as much as I used to.
I notice I am losing weight.
I have trouble with constipation.
My heart beats faster than usual.
I feel hopeful about the future.
I find it easy to make decisions.

There are four choices of response category, with numerical values of 1–4: a little of the time; some of the time; a good part of the time; most of the time.

Scoring

Each item scores 1–4. The score values for the 20 items are summed. An index is derived by dividing the sum of the raw scores by the maximum possible score of 80, converted to a decimal and multiplied by 100 (Zung et al. 1965).

Zung et al. (1965) reported that the mean score on the Zung Scale for outpatients diagnosed as depressive reaction was 64. Zung (1965) reported that the mean score for hospitalized in-patients diagnosed with depressive disorders was 74.

Validity

Zung et al. (1965) tested the scale for validity using the Minnesota

Multiphasic Personality Inventory as a gold standard. They administered the scale to new psychiatric out-patients at Duke University (number not specified). The correlations between their instrument and three sub-scales of the Minnesota Inventory were: 0.70, 0.68 and 0.13. The authors commented that the latter correlation was 'unexpectedly low'. Brown and Zung (1972) tested the scale against the Hamilton Depression Scale and reported a correlation of 0.79.

The scale is also able to distinguish between patients with a confirmed diagnosis of a depressive state and patients with an initial diagnosis of depression, but subsequently reviewed and given another psychiatric diagnosis (Zung 1965; 1967). Zung et al. (1965) reported the scale was able to distinguish reliably between patients with a psychoneurotic depression and those with an anxiety reaction and found the instrument sensitive to clinical change. However, Toner et al. (1988) reported that the convergent validity of the Zung scale with physicians' judgements was lower than that of the well-tested Comprehensive Assessment and Referral Evaluation (CARE) scale, 0.65 (Kappa: 0.29) in comparison with 0.73 (Kappa: 0.46). Arfwidsson et al. (1974) cast doubt on the validity of the scale, suggesting that doctors' ratings are more valid as a means of assessing the degree and quality of depressive symptoms. Also, Carroll et al. (1973) assessed patients known to have varying degrees of depression and reported that the Zung scale was unable to distinguish between the groups; they reported a correlation of 0.41 between interview-based and Zung ratings. Carroll et al. blame the self-report method rather than the Zung scale, as the former adopts a different perspective to a psychiatric interviewer. Other studies have found the Zung scale to be unresponsive to changes in treatment patterns (Hamilton 1976).

Reliability

There is little evidence of the scale's reliability. The scale has been used successfully with clustering techniques by Byrne (1978). Also, response rates for self-completed scales may be lower than for administered scales. A comparative study of Zung's scale with the short version of CARE showed a response rate of 65 per cent for Zung and 100 per cent for CARE. Among the reasons for non-response were visual problems (28 per cent), illiteracy (9 per cent) and lack of motivation (34 per cent) (Toner et al. 1988). These response difficulties apply to all self-rating scales.

Montgomery–Asberg Depression Rating Scale

The Montgomery–Asberg Depression Rating Scale was developed by Montgomery and Asberg (1979) on the basis of 54 English and 52 Swedish patients who completed a 65-item psychopathology scale. Analysis identified the 17 most commonly occurring symptoms in depressive illness in the sample. Subsequent analyses, using 64 patients on different types of antidepressive drugs, were then used to create a 10-item depression scale which consisted of those items showing the greatest changes with treatment.

This scale is oriented toward psychic symptoms and covers apparent sadness, reported sadness, inability to feel, difficulty in concentration, inner tension, pessimistic thoughts, suicidal thoughts, lassitude, reduced sleep and reduced appetite. The scale's advantage lies in its brevity.

Content

The scale's ten items encompass the most commonly occurring symptoms of depressive illness which change in response to treatment (see above). Examples are:

Apparent sadness: representing despondency, gloom and despair (more than just ordinary transient low spirits), reflected in speech, facial expression and posture. Rate by depth and Inability to brighten up:

0 No sadness.
1
2 Looks dispirited but does brighten up without difficulty.
3
4 Appears sad and unhappy most of the time.
5
6 Looks miserable all the time. Extremely despondent.

Reduced sleep: representing the experience of reduced duration or depth of sleep compared to the subject's own normal pattern when well.

0 Sleeps as usual.
1
2 Slight difficulty dropping off to sleep or slightly reduced, light or fitful sleep.
3
4 Sleep reduced or broken up by at least two hours.
5
6 Less than two or three hours' sleep.

Lassitude: representing a difficulty getting started or slowness initiating and performing everyday activities.

0 Hardly any difficulty in getting started. No sluggishness.
1 Difficulties in starting activities.
2
3
4 Difficulties in starting simple routine activities which are carried out with effort.
5
6 Complete lassitude. Unable to do anything without help.

Pessimistic thoughts: representing thoughts of guilt, inferiority, self-reproach, sinfulness, remorse and ruin.

0 No pessimistic thoughts.
1
2 Fluctuating ideas of failure, self-reproach or self-depreciation.
3
4 Persistent self-accusation, or definite but still rational ideas of guilt or sin. Increasingly pessimistic about the future.
5
6 Delusions of ruin, remorse or unredeemable sin. Self-accusations which are absurd and unshakeable.

Scoring

Scoring involves computing of scale items. The procedure of arriving at a definition of a case by adding up numbers derived from a severity-grade score of a number of symptoms has a certain attraction until it is realized that one case may be very different from another.

Validity

Montgomery and Asberg (1979) tested scale scores against psychiatrists' judgements, using 18 patients who responded to treatment and 17 who did not. The scale was able to discriminate between the two groups. The scale was also tested against the Hamilton Rating Scale with a reported correlation of 0.70.

The sensitivity of the scale is questionable. Cooper and Fairburn (1986) found that a group of bulimic and a group of depressed patients had similar scores on the Montgomery–Asberg Depression Rating Scale but different symptoms, or scale items, contributed strongly to the overall score in the two groups.

Reliability

Good results for reliability have been reported by the authors and the scale was found to be robust when used by different professionals in a variety of health-care settings (GPs, nurses, psychologists, psychiatrists) and high inter-rater correlations were produced. Comparisons between two English raters, two Swedish raters and one English and one Swedish rater, rating 11 to 30 patients, produced correlations of between 0.89 and 0.97.

However, 30 per cent of the total score is apparently accounted for by three items which all commonly occur in physical illnesses and states of distress other than depression (Williams 1984; Cooper and Fairburn 1986).

In sum, the scale items and the scoring procedure question the reliability of the scale.

Hamilton Depression Scale

This is a widely used observer scale which includes assessment of cognitive and behavioural components of depression and is particularly thorough in the assessment of the somatic aspects (Hamilton 1967). Like many depression scales, the Hamilton Depression Scale cannot be used to establish a diagnosis of depression, but only to assess severity once depression has already been diagnosed. Interviewer training is required.

Content

The Hamilton Depression Scale (Hamilton 1959; 1967) consists of 21 items: depressed mood, feelings of guilt, suicidal ideation, work and activities, insight, retardation, agitation, insomnia (early, middle and late), psychic anxiety, somatic anxiety, gastro-intestinal symptoms, general somatic symptoms, genital symptoms (loss of libido or menstrual disturbances), hypochondriases and loss of weight. Examples of scale items are:

Depressed mood: 0–4

Gloomy attitude, pessimism about the future
Feeling of sadness
Tendency to weep:
   sadness and/or mild depression
   occasional weeping and/or moderate depression
   frequent weeping and/or severe depression
   extreme symptoms

Anxiety, psychic: 0–4

Tension and irritability
Worrying about minor matters
Apprehensive attitude
Fears

Somatic symptoms, gastrointestinal: 0–2

Loss of appetite
Heavy feelings in abdomen
Constipation

Insight: 0–2

Loss of insight
Partial or doubtful loss
No loss

The somatic categories of the scale have been used alone, in conjunction with other depression-rating scales. The somatic items relate to muscular, sensory systems and to cardiovascular, respiratory, gastro-intestinal, genito-urinary and autonomic symptoms. For example Martin (1987) used these items without the Hamilton depression (psychosomatic) items together with the Montgomery–Asberg Depression Rating Scale.

Scoring

Some items are scored 0–4 and others are scored 0–2. Scale items marked 0–4 have the response choices for the rater of absent (0), mild or trivial (1), moderate (2–3), severe (4); and scale items marked 0–2 have the choice of absent (0), slight or doubtful (1), clearly present (2). The items are individually scored by a rater during an interview. The interpretation of categories is described by Hamilton (1967) and reproduced by Williams (1984).

The total scores range from 0–100 (representing the sum of two raters' scores or double the score for one rater). Some studies report total scores with a maximum of 50.

Validity

The scale is reported to have high concurrent validity with good agreement with other scales, particularly the Beck, with correlations reported of over 0.70 (Hamilton 1976). Carroll et al. (1973) reported that the Hamilton scale was better able than the Beck Depression Inventory to distinguish between groups of patients known to have varying degrees of depression. They argued that self-report scales, such as the Beck, over-weight subjective scores. Hamilton (1967) reported that the scale discriminated between men and women; women generally are more likely to have higher depression scores than men.

Reliability

Its inter-rater reliability is reported to be good: correlations are high ranging from 0.84 to 0.90 (see reviews by Hamilton 1976 and Rehm 1981). However, six of the scale items are symptoms of somatic disturbance and account for 31 per cent of the possible total score; if the insomnia items which so often rate highly in physical illness are included, then 42 per cent of the total is accounted for (Williams 1984).

Although popular, the scale should be viewed with caution, given the number of items measuring somatic problems.

The Beck Depression Inventory (BDI)

If the researcher is interested only in depression, and not more generally in both anxiety and depression, then it is reasonable to use a specially designed scale. The Beck Depression Inventory (BDI) is such a specific scale. It was designed by Beck *et al.* (1961) and is widely used. It was designed because other widely used scales (e.g. the Minnesota Multiphasic Personality Inventory) were not specifically designed for the measurement of depression or were based on old psychiatric nomenclature. It was developed on the basis of the authors' observations of samples of 226 and 183 depressed patients' attitudes and symptoms while undergoing psychotherapy. These observations led to the creation of a 21-item inventory; each category describes a specific behavioural manifestation of depression and consists of a series of self-evaluation items which are graded and ranked according to severity (neutral to maximum). A 13-item version of the scale has also been developed (Reynolds and Gould 1981).

The Beck Depression Inventory is generally regarded as better than the Minnesota Multiphasic Personality Inventory and better than similar scales such as the Zung scale (Hammen 1981). Originally developed to be interviewer administered, it is now a self-rating scale. A large proportion of items relate to somatic disturbance, and this has led to some controversy.

Like the Hamilton, it cannot be used to diagnose depression in the absence of a prior diagnosis – it is only a measure of severity once the clinical diagnosis has been made. This is to exclude people being diagnosed as depressed when they have high BDI scores for situational reasons (e.g. bereavement). It has been reported to have acceptable levels of reliability for use as a research screening instrument with an elderly population (Gallagher *et al.* 1982).

Content

The BDI consists of 21 items, each with 4 response choices, in the form of statements, ranked in order of severity, from which the respondent selects one that best fits the way s/he feels at 'this moment'. The symptoms and attitudes which the scale aims to measure are sadness, pessimism/discouragement, sense of failure, dissatisfaction, guilt, expectation of punishment, self-dislike, self-accusation, suicidal ideation, crying, irritability, social withdrawal, indecisiveness, body-image distortion, work retardation, insomnia, fatiguability, anorexia, weight loss, somatic preoccupation and loss of libido. Examples of items, are:

I am not particularly pessimistic or discouraged about the future.
I feel I have nothing to look forward to.
I feel that I won't ever get over my troubles.
I feel that the future is hopeless and that things cannot improve.

I am no more irritated now than I ever am.
I get annoyed or irritated more easily than I used to.
I feel irritated all the time.
I don't get irritated at all by the things that used to irritate me.

I have not lost interest in other people.
I am less interested in other people now than I used to be.
I have lost most of my interest in other people and have little feeling for them.
I have lost all my interest in other people and don't care about them at all.

Scoring

The Beck Depression Inventory is based on a Guttman scale. The original scale permitted selections of four to seven responses which were given a weight of 0 to 3. Revisions to the scale were made in 1974 and in 1978, standardizing the response choices to four for each item; each still carries a weight of 0 to 3.

The numerical values of 0 to 3 which are assigned to each statement indicate the degree of severity. In some categories two alternative statements (2a and 2b) are presented at a given level but are assigned the same weight. Items are scored, with a maximum total of 63. Normative data suggest the following categories of severity level: normal 0–9; mild 10–15; mild–moderate 16–19; moderate–severe 20–29; severe > 29. The BDI is available in a format suitable for computer scoring from National Computer Systems, Minneapolis.

Validity

The scale correlates well with clinicians' ratings of severity of depression and with other depression scales. Beck et al. (1961), on the basis of 226 hospital out-patients and admissions, and 183 patients in a replication group, tested the BDI against independent psychiatric diagnoses made by four psychiatrists. Their agreement with the scale was 56 per cent; and agreement within one degree of specificity was achieved in 97 per cent of cases. The authors reported that the scale was able to discriminate between depth-of-depression categories based on clinical ratings for both original and replication groups, the correlations ranging from 0.59 to 0.68. Correlations of 0.66 were obtained between the Beck and Depression Adjective Check Lists and of 0.75 with the Beck and the Minnesota Multiphasic Personality Inventory (Beck 1970). It has been used successfully in clinical and general populations, although most studies have focused on psychiatric patients (Beck et al. 1961; Williams 1984). It correlates moderately to highly with the Hamilton Rating Scale (Hamilton 1976), although Carroll et al. (1973) argue that this camouflages the lack of congruence at severe levels of depression. A review of the literature from 1961 to 1986 by Beck et al. (1988) reported that the concurrent validities of the BDI with respect to comparisons with clinical ratings and the Hamilton Scale for Depression were high. The mean correlations with the Hamilton Scale and clinical ratings for psychiatric patients were over 0.70. The respective mean correlations for non-psychiatric patients were 0.74 and 0.60. The Beck was also shown to discriminate between sub-types of depression and to distinguish depression from anxiety. The literature reviewed indicated relationships with the Beck and suicidal behaviour and alcoholism. The scale has been reported to be associated with perceived social support in a study of carers for elderly confused people (those with lower BDI scores reported that they received greater social support) (Morris et al. 1989). The literature reviewed by Beck et al. (1988) also suggests that the BDI represents one underlying general syndrome of depression, comprising three highly intercorrelated factors: negative attitudes to self, performance impairment and somatic disturbance.

Reliability

Reliability was tested by the authors on the basis of 226 hospital out-patients and admissions and 183 patients in a replication group (all adults). Internal consistency was tested using 200 of the cases. The score for each of the 21 items was tested with the total BDI score for each person; all were associated at the $P < 0.0001$ level. Split-half reliability was tested using 97 of the cases, the correlation between the two halves of the scale was 0.86. Split-half reliability was also assessed using a group of adults by Weckowicz et al. (1967); these authors reported a lower figure of 0.53.

Beck et al. (1961) carried out test-retest correlations, along with repeated psychiatric ratings in case people remembered their scores or genuinely changed between testings. Consistent relationships between the instrument and clinical ratings were reported, using 38 cases, at two- to five-week intervals. Reliability coefficients were above 0.90. (Beck et al. 1961; Beck 1970). Test-retest correlations at 6 and 21 days apart were also carried out by Gallagher et al. (1982) on a sample of 159 patients and volunteers from a 'senior centre' in Los Angeles. Test-retest correlations for the total sample, the normal sub-sample and the depressed sub-sample were: 0.90, 0.86 and 0.79 respectively. They also carried out tests for the internal consistency of the scale and reported coefficient alphas of 0.91, 0.76 and 0.73 for these three groups respectively. The extensive review of the literature by Beck *et al.* (1988) reported that a meta-analysis of the BDI's internal consistency estimates yielded a mean coefficient alpha of 0.86 for psychiatric patients and 0.81 for non-psychiatric respondents.

Tests to data indicate that the scale has moderate to good levels of validity and reliability, although most testing has been conducted on psychiatric populations. It is regarded as the scale of choice for researchers in the selection of depressed subjects from a larger population, although, as with most scales, its accuracy depends on subjects' motivation to report their emotional state accurately (Stehouwer 1985). A comprehensive review of the literature on the reliability and validity of the scale has been published by Beck *et al.* (1988).

Hospital Anxiety and Depression Scale (HAD)

The Hospital Anxiety and Depression Scale was developed by Zigmond and Snaith (1983). It is a brief assessment of anxiety and depression, consisting of 14 items divided into two subscales for anxiety and depression, in which the patient rates each item on a 4-point scale.

Two common problems with questionnaires for the detection of mood disorders are that scores are affected by the physical illness of the patient, and there is insufficient distinction between one mood disorder and another. Zigmond and Snaith developed the Hospital Anxiety and Depression Scale in partial response to this. The scale measures anhedonic depression which the authors take as the best indicator of hypomelancholia and advise the prescription of anti-depressants for those with a high score. Snaith (1987) also recommends the use of a combined researcher-administered and self-assessment scale.

The authors purposefully excluded all items relating to both emotional and physical disorder (e.g. dizziness, headaches), and the items included in the HAD were based solely on the psychic symptoms of neurosis. They also aimed to distinguish between the concepts of anxiety and depression. The 8 items comprising the depression subscale were based on the anhedonic state. The authors justified this by reference to the evidence that this is probably the central psychopathological feature of that form of depression which responds well to antidepressant drug treatment and is therefore clinically useful information. The 8 items comprising the anxiety subscale were selected after study of the Present State Examination and analysis of the psychic manifestations of anxiety neurosis. Severity scales were developed, with ratings from 0 to 3.

Content

Unlike most other scales, the HAD is not derived from factor analysis but from clinical experience. It consists of two sections, with 4-point response scales. The scale assesses emotional state over the 'past week'. Examples of the scale are:

I feel tense or 'wound up':
Most of the time.
A lot of the time.
From time to time, occasionally.

Worrying thoughts go through my mind:
A great deal of the time.
A lot of the time.
From time to time but not too often.
Only occasionally.

I feel as if I am slowed down:
Nearly all the time.
Very often.
Sometimes.
Not at all.

I get sudden feelings of panic:
Very often indeed.
Quite often.
Not very often.
Not at all.

Scoring

Individual items are scored from 0–3 to 3–0, depending on the direction of the item wording. The higher scores indicate the presence of problems. Using psychiatric diagnoses as a gold standard, HAD depression ratings of 7 or less were considered to be non-cases; scores of 8–10 were considered doubtful cases; and scores of 11+ implies definite cases.

Validity

The scales were tested for validity on over 100 psychiatric out-patients and hospital staff, with good results (Zigmond and Snaith 1983).

In relation to sensitivity, further tests showed that physically ill patients, who were not assessed as having mood disorder, had similar scores to the normal sample and scale scores were judged not to be affected by physical illness.

Reliability

Attempts were made to overcome response bias in the scale by alternating the order of responses so that at one item the first response indicates maximum severity and at another item the last response indicates maximum severity. Four possible responses were chosen to prevent people from opting for a middle grade.

The authors tested internal consistency of the scale, using data from 50 patients. The correlations for the anxiety items ranged from 0.76 to 0.41. The analysis of the depression items revealed one weak item which was removed from the scale ('I am awake before I need to get up'), along with the weakest of the anxiety items. The remaining depression items had correlations ranging from 0.60 to 0.30.

The criteria were then tested for reliability with a further 50 patients and results judged to be satisfactory (the false positive/negative rates were between 1 and 5 per cent). The severity ratings correlated with psychiatric judgements, with the results for depression: 0.70, and for anxiety: 0.74. Correlations between items and interviewer ratings provided some evidence that the depression and anxiety items were tapping different mood dimensions, rather than the same thing, although some overlap is inevitable. It was apparently easily understood and completed by patients.

Although the authors present the HAD as a reliable and valid instrument on the basis of these tests, far more work on its reliability and validity is required to be carried out before its performance as an indicator can be confidently judged.

The Symptoms of Anxiety and Depression Scale (SAD)

The Symptoms of Anxiety and Depression Scale assesses anxiety and depression by focusing exclusively on recent symptomatology 'within the last month'. It is a brief self-report measure, empirically derived from two other scales developed by the authors (Bedford *et al.* 1976).

The SAD has been adapted for use with the elderly (McNab and Phillip, 1980). McNab and Phillip (1980) reported their study using the SAD in which 41 people aged 85 and over were visited by health visitors based in one group general practice. The questions were apparently well tolerated by respondents. They reported that 80.5 per cent scored within the normal range, 17.1 per cent were borderline and 2.4 per cent were ill. These scores did not differ significantly from those reported for younger adults by Bedford *et al.* (1976).

Results from Vetter *et al.*'s (1982) study of 1,288 people aged 70+ living at home in Wales are broadly consistent with others. They report borderline anxiety in 19 per cent of respondents, and pathological scores in 7 per cent.

Females had a higher degree of anxiety than males, although there was no consistent variation of anxiety score with age. In relation to depression, 6 per cent achieved a borderline score and 3 per cent pathological scores. Females again scored higher than males, and there was no consistent variation with age.

Content

The scale consists of seven states of anxiety and seven states of depression. Examples of items, which relate to 'the past week or so', are:

Recently, have you been worried about every little thing?
Recently, have you been so worked up that you couldn't keep still?
Recently, have you had a pain or tense feeling in the back of your neck?
Recently, has worry kept you awake at night?
Recently, have you lost interest in just about everything?

All items responses are 'no/a little/a lot/unbearably'.

Scoring

For each question a score of 0–3 is possible, rated according to the degree of distress (none = 0, a little = 1, a lot = 2, unbearably = 3). The scores are added for the seven questions at each of the two measures, giving a range of 0–21 for each scale, and 0–42 overall.

By comparison with psychiatric opinion, psychiatrically normal scores are judged to be those section SAD scores of 0–2; 3–5 were regarded as borderline; and 6–21 as pathological, indicating extreme dysphoria or clinically significant depression.

Validity

There is some work on the construct and predictive validity of the scale. The SAD has been used recently by Morgan et al. (1987) in a survey of 979 people aged 65+ living at home in Nottinghamshire. The authors reported a relationship between physical- and mental-health problems, and that emotional disturbance increased the likelihood of medical consultations. However, they also reported a weak correlation between SAD scores and clinical ratings of depression (0.43), and between the SAD and clinical ratings of the severity of depression (0.32). In contrast, Bedford et al. (1976), in tests involving 96 in-patients rated by psychiatrists and psychologists, reported a statistically significant association between patients' depression scores and psychiatrists' ratings of their depression levels.

McNab and Phillip (1980), in their study of people aged 85+, reported that respondents' SAD scores did not differ significantly from health-visitor ratings of the same respondents' mental health, although the degree of concordance was reported to be modest at best.

Vetter and Ford (1989) also used the scale in Wales to predict falls among elderly people and reported a relationship between scale score and the prevalence of falls. On the other hand, as this study was cross-sectional, the long-term predictive ability of the scale was not tested.

Little other published work on its validation exists.

Reliability

Bedford *et al.* (1976) reported test-retest results at one month for 68 (out of 96 initially rated) patients rated by psychiatrists and psychologists using the SAD scale. The results showed evidence of a significant change, from an average score of 12.68 to 6.40. The authors cite this change as evidence of its sensitivity to change in mental state rather than as unreliability. Split-half reliability correlations were 0.61 for normal control subjects and 0.69 for the patients.

Again, evidence is scant on its reliability. In sum, although this is an increasingly popular scale for use with elderly populations, far more extensive testing is required before it can be generally recommended.

The General Health Questionnaire (GHQ)

The General Health Questionnaire is the most widely applied measure of psychiatric disturbance in the UK and also has numerous worldwide applications. A major advantage for potential users of the GHQ is the existence of periodically updated handbooks containing its method, a comprehensive review of applications, and studies of reliability and validity (Goldberg 1978; Goldberg and Williams 1988).

The GHQ was developed in London during the 1960s and 1970s and was intended for use in general practice settings. It was derived from various scales, including the Cornell Medical Index. In the construction of the GHQ the concept of psychiatric disorder was thought to be appropriate to general practice settings.

The GHQ is a screening questionnaire for detecting independently verifiable forms of psychiatric illness and does not make clinical diagnoses. If these are necessary, a two-stage strategy must be employed. It is not suitable for the assessment of long-stage (chronic) problems, as it does not detect them. It is a pure state measure, assessing present state in relation to usual state (this question wording is not distortive as most people see their usual state as a normal state) (Goldberg and Williams 1988).

The advantage of the GHQ is that it concentrates on broader components of psychiatric morbidity (particularly anxiety and depression) and is designed to be self-administered. It does not attempt to detect mental subnormality, senile dementia or mania (most of the people within these categories would not be able to complete the questionnaire). It was not intended to be used for the detection of functional psychoses (schizophrenia or psychotic depression), although these conditions are in fact detected. A study of 111 acute geriatric medical in-patients by O'Riordan *et al.* (1990) showed that there were no significant differences on the GHQ when dementia was the variable (e.g. between normal depressed patients and demented depressed patients), although threshold scores did require raising.

One further advantage of using the GHQ is that short-item versions exist (12, 20, 28, 30), which, although slightly less valid and sensitive than the long version (60 items), are more suitable than the longer versions for use with older frail people. The 28-item version has an additional advantage over the other versions in that it also permits analysis within sub-categories; it was developed mainly for research purposes.

There have been numerous applications of the GHQ in survey research and in clinical settings (e.g. GPs' surgeries). More recently it has been used among 662 people aged 85 and over living in London and was found to be acceptable to respondents, although some required assistance with completion due to poor sight and stiff finger joints (Bowling 1990).

Although it has been used extensively in the UK, there have also been many applications of the scale in other countries, particularly in the USA. The 30-item version, for example, was used in a psychological morbidity survey of 1,649 new adult enrollers in a Health Maintenance Organization in the USA (Berwick *et al.* 1987).

Although the GHQ is culture specific in development, it works well in other settings, e.g. among both white and black residents in Philadelphia, in Calcutta, China, rural Iceland, Brazil and Australia (Tennant 1977; Mari and Williams 1985; for review see Goldberg and Williams 1988). It has been translated into at least 38 languages.

Content

The original version of the GHQ consists of 60 items; shorter versions of 30, 28, 20 and 12 have also been developed. The 12-item version is apparently as efficient as the 30-item version as a case detector.

Examples of questions, which relate to the past few weeks, are:

Have you recently:

Been able to concentrate on whatever you're doing?

Better than usual, same as usual, less than usual, much less than usual.

Spent much time chatting with people?

More time than usual, about the same as usual, less time than usual, much less than usual.

Felt on the whole you were doing things well?

Better than usual, about the same, less well than usual, much less well.

Been feeling unhappy and depressed?

Not at all, no more than usual, rather more than usual, much more than usual.

Felt that life isn't worth living?

Not at all, no more than usual, rather more than usual, much more than usual.

Scoring

The GHQ consists of a check-list of statements asking respondents to compare their recent experience to their usual state on a 4-point scale of severity. The scoring scale consists of 0 or 1 (the 0–0–1–1 scoring scale, the scores following the sequence of response categories across the page from left to right, is the most commonly used). Some items are negative, others are positive. The overall GHQ is the sum of the item scores. The 0–0–1–1 scoring scale is simply a count of the symptoms and is the simplest and also avoids the problems of middle-user response bias. Goldberg and Williams (1988) demonstrated that very similar results are obtained with the different scoring methods in existence, and little is gained by a Likert severity score.

Threshold scores are defined as equivalent to the concept of 'caseness' that corresponds to the average patient referred to psychiatrists. If the results of a population of GHQ scores are compared with independent psychiatric assessment, it is possible to state the number of symptoms where the probability that an individual will be thought to be a case exceeds 0.5. This is called a threshold score. The proportion of respondents with scores above this threshold is the probable prevalence of illness. Finlay-Jones and Murphy (1979) have shown that in order to identify 'cases' that correspond to standards derived from the Present State Examination, it is necessary to raise the threshold score.

Since physically ill people score highly on the GHQ, it is not surprising that they are overrepresented among false positives. Goldberg and Williams suggest raising the thresholds for use with severe physical illnesses. Goldberg (1978), in the manual for the administration of the GHQ, points to the necessity of manipulating the threshold score to enhance discrimination in different populations.

It is possible to compare the amount of psychiatric disturbance in two populations by comparison of the central tendency (mean, median) and dispersion (SD, inter-quartile range) of scores in each population. Also a given population can be tested on different occasions to assess the changes in psychiatric disturbance over time.

Because of the nature of its response scale, the GHQ is likely to miss very long standing disorders, since respondents answer 'same as usual' (and thus score zero) for symptoms they are experiencing and have been experiencing for a long time. However, Goldberg and Williams (1988) point out that the loss of cases is minimal as many people cling to a concept of their 'usual self' as being without symptoms. They suggest including questions on medication taking and whether the person thinks s/he has a nervous illness to detect chronic patients. However, Goodchild and Duncan Jones (1985) have suggested an ingenious scoring method which may increase the sensitivity of the GHQ and makes it more likely to detect long-standing illness. This consists of dividing the GHQ items up into items detecting caseness (negative, e.g. feeling constantly under strain) and those indicating health (positive, e.g. enjoying day-to-day activities). This method assigns a score to those replying 'same as usual' to any of the negative items (so the score for negative items becomes 0111, and for positive items 0011). This method gives superior validity coefficients against caseness over the normal GHQ scoring method (0011) as measured by the Present State Examination. A further advantage is that the scores are more normally distributed and the scale is a more sensitive indicator when used over time. Given the recent development of this method, Goldberg and Williams suggest that this method should be used in addition to previous methods, rather than instead of.

Validity

There is good evidence that assessments of the severity of psychiatric illness are directly proportional to the number of symptoms reported on the GHQ (Goldberg and Huxley 1980). The predictive validity of the GHQ in comparison with other well-known scaling tests of depression is also good (Goldberg 1985; Williams 1987).

The principal components and item analysis used during the development of the GHQ ensured that it has content validity; its construct validity was demonstrated in the principal components analysis which showed that there was a large general factor found in all the analyses reported.

Berwick et al. (1987) carried out a factor analysis of responses which disclosed six factors (anxiety/strain, confidence, depression, energy, social function and insomnia) and a strong tendency for items of similar wording (positive phrasing) to cluster together.

Over 50 validity studies have been conducted of the GHQ. Although not perfect, it correlates well with psychiatric diagnoses of morbidity and depression (Finlay-Jones and Murphy 1979; Williams 1987). The GHQ-30 has been the most widely validated. For example, 29 such studies were reported by Goldberg and Williams (1988). Correlations with other gold standards have established the criterion validity of the GHQ. Using standardized psychiatric interviews as a gold standard, reported sensitivities range between 0.55 and 0.92, and specificities between 0.80 and 0.99, depending on the choice of threshold score (Vieweg and Hedlund 1983). Comparisons of GHQ scores with a structured clinical interview (e.g. the Present State Examination or the Clinical Interview Schedule) report correlations from 0.45 to 0.83. The GHQ-60 had the highest correlations and the GHQ-30 the poorest (see Goldberg and Williams 1988 for review).

Also a study in the USA found a correlation of 0.72 between the Beck Depression Index and the GHQ-30 (Cavanaugh 1983), and an Australian study reported a correlation of 0.57 between the Zung depression scales and the 30-item GHQ (Henderson et al. 1981). Bowling and Browne (1991), on the basis of surveys with 662 people aged 85+ and almost 800 aged 65+ living at home in London and in Essex, reported correlations with the GHQ and Neugarten's Life Satisfaction Scale A of 0.47 in each case (Essex data is unpublished). This is a moderate correlation, reflecting the different dimensions of emotional well-being tapped by these two scales. Watson and Evans (1986), in their study of the health of a multi-cultural sample of mothers with young children in London's East End, reported that mothers' GHQ scores correlated well with interviewers' ratings of the mothers' distress. A further application was undertaken more recently by Jenkinson et al. (1988). The 30-item GHQ and the Nottingham Health Profile (NHP) were administered to people suffering from either migraine or arthritis. Correlations between the emotional-reactions subsection of the NHP and the GHQ were moderate (0.49) for both groups of patients.

Although the GHQ was not developed as a predictive tool, some studies have reported findings demonstrating predictive validity, although two studies have reported negative results. Criterion validity was established using health services as the criterion. Those with the highest GHQ scores have been reported to have the highest use of services (e.g. general practitioner services) (Goldberg and Williams 1988). Berwick et al. (1987) provided further evidence of the predictive validity of the GHQ:

elevations of GHQ scores, over two administrations at 7-month intervals, were strongly associated with the probability of both mental-health and non-mental-health care within twelve months of enrolment.

The GHQ is sensitive for transient disorders, detecting symptoms of at least two weeks' duration. It is as sensitive to depression disorders as any of the specially designed depression scales (such as the Beck or HAD) and detects anxiety disorders as well, so it is suitable for use when the researcher wants a broader measure. Numerous surveys indicate that the GHQ is suitable for use with younger and older men and women in community and primary health care settings (Sims and Salmons 1975; Tarnopolsky et al. 1979; Benjamin et al. 1982; Cleary et al. 1982; Banks 1983; Hobbs et al. 1983; 1984; Goldberg and Williams 1988).

Another example of the application of the GHQ was by Watson and Evans (1986) with a multi-cultural sample of mothers with young children. They found that mothers' GHQ scores correlated well with interviewers' ratings of the mothers' distress. An analysis of the translation of the questionnaire into Bengali for the Bengali mothers did reveal some problems. The questionnaire was back-translated by an independent translator. There was a high level of agreement between one translation and the original, with the exception of the item: 'Have you recently been feeling nervous and strung up all the time?' which was translated as 'Did you suffer from mental breakdown and mental anxiety?' The other translation had problems with the item 'Have you recently been finding life a struggle all the time?' which was translated 'Are you thinking yourself a struggler?'

They also found that not all items were applicable to mothers with young babies, e.g. 'Have you recently been having restless disturbed nights?'; 'Have you been getting out of the house as much as usual?'; 'Have you spent much time chatting with people?' Because young mothers are more likely to have false positive scores with these items, the authors recommend raising the threshold score, using the 30-item version, from 4 or 5 to 8.

There can be other problems in administration which may affect reliability. Very elderly people with failing eyesight and arthritic fingers may have difficulty completing the GHQ independently and will require varying degrees of assistance from an interviewer (e.g. reading out the items or recording responses). It is unknown whether this produces any social desirability bias; this is a problem potentially affecting all self-rating scales (Bowling 1990).

Reliability

Split-half and test-retest correlations have been carried out on the GHQ with good results. Split-half reliability has been carried out with 853 completed questionnaires, and the correlation achieved was 0.95. Internal consistency, using Cronbach's alpha, has been reported in a range of studies with correlations ranging from 0.77 to −0.93. Test-retest reliability correlations have been reported ranging from 0.51 to 0.90, the correlations being higher with clinically defined groups with a high prevalence of disorder (Goldberg and Williams 1988). A problem posed by test-retest reliability is one of distinguishing between true change and unreliability. Goldberg and Williams state that the definitive test-retest reliability study of the GHQ remains to be done.

The Geriatric Mental State (GMS)

The problem of recognizing depression in the elderly is exacerbated because it may present with features similar to dementia; the two conditions may also co-exist. This has led to many researchers in psychiatry turning to instruments of high validity and reliability in relation to the elderly, e.g. the Comprehensive Assessment and Referral Evaluation interview schedule (CARE) (Gurland, 1980) and the Geriatric Mental State Examination (Henderson et al. 1983).

Copeland et al. (1976) reported the development of the Geriatric Mental State (GMS) which was derived from British and US instruments: the Present State Examination (PSE) devised by Wing et al. (1974) and the Psychiatric Status Schedule (Spitzer et al. 1970). They scaled this down to a form suitable for use in community settings, and they used it within a broader semi-structured interview schedule called the Comprehensive Assessment and Referral Evaluation (CARE) interview (Gurland et al. 1983; Copeland et al. 1978; 1987b). The CARE interview is broad and covers psychiatric, medical, nutritional, economic and social problems. Interviewer training is required for CARE and for the GMS.

The psychiatric diagnosis derived from the GMS has since been standardized by the application of computer methods and called AGECAT (Dewey and Copeland 1986). AGECAT was used on a sample of general practitioners' elderly patients in Liverpool and produced diagnosis of depressive neurosis in 8 per cent of cases, and of depressive psychosis of 3 per cent (total 11 per cent). If marginal cases were included, the incidence of mild depression was 22 per cent which was close to the 20 per cent found in the early study in Newcastle (Kay et al. 1964; Copeland et al. 1987a; 1987b).

The GMS is a well-validated and tested scale but is extremely lengthy, although there is a shorter community version available (GMSA), which is still fairly lengthy if used alongside a survey questionnaire. The short version was developed on the basis of data from a random sample of 396 elderly people living at home in London. The full length GMS is frequently used as a gold standard against which to assess other scales of mental state; it has been chosen as the principal instrument in the three Medical Research Council multi-site studies ongoing in the UK and in three similar studies initiated by the World Health and Pan-American Health Organizations (Copeland 1990).

The full GMS takes between 30 and 45 minutes to administer. The CARE, which has 1,500 items concerned with expressed physical symptoms, social problems and the use of services, takes between one and a half to two hours. The short community version (GMSA) takes from 15–20 minutes.

Since 1976 the GMS has been translated into French, Spanish, German, Danish, Dutch and Icelandic. There have been a number of applications of the GMS. The authors of the instrument have also published a number of papers based on analyses of their studies using the GMS (Copeland *et al.* 1986; Dewey and Copeland 1986; Copeland *et al.* 1987a; 1987b; 1988; Davidson *et al.* 1988; Sullivan *et al.* 1988; McWilliam *et al.* 1988; Saunders *et al.* 1989).

Content

The GMS consists of standard tests and interviewer ratings of the degree of confidence in the information. The confusion items are standard (e.g. checks on day of week). Examples of other items are:

Guilt
Do you tend to blame yourself for anything or feel guilty about anything? What?
Code: Obvious self-blame over past and present peccadilloes.
Mentions regrets about past which may or may not be justifiable

Irritability
Have you been more irritable (angry) lately?
Code: Admits to irritability (anger).

Concentration
Can you concentrate on a television (radio, film) programme? Can you watch it (listen to it) all the way through?
Code: difficulty in concentrating on entertainment.

Perceptual distortion
Is something odd (strange) going on which you cannot explain?
Code: Puzzled by something odd going on.

Scoring

Detailed instructions on the rating, coding and scoring procedures, which are fairly lengthy, are available from the authors in the Department of Psychiatry at the University of Liverpool.

Validity

The full CARE interview has been tested against psychiatric judgements on 396 subjects in Greater London, with high overall agreement: agreement on depression and dementia reached 88 per cent of cases (Cohen's kappa for overall agreement was 0.7) and AGECAT (a computerized diagnostic system) was judged to provide a reasonable diagnosis (Copeland *et al.* 1986). Equally good agreement levels were patient knowing s/he is being tested, and the other half can follow after *et al.* 1987a; 1987b).

The convergent validity of the Zung scale with physicians' judgements was lower than that achieved by CARE, 0.65 (Kappa: 0.29), in comparison with 0.73 (Kappa: 0.46) (Toner *et al.* 1988).

Reliability

Reliability studies were initially undertaken in London and New York, and in Australia and Liverpool with the shorter versions. Inter-rater reliability was 69 per cent for the first study but only 38 per cent in the second, although partial agreement was much higher at between 80 and 85 per cent. No significant differences in the number of positive ratings made between interviewers in the US or UK were found. In the Australian study, Henderson *et al.* (1983) reported satisfactory inter-rater reliability of the shortened version with average correlations of 0.56 and 0.84.

The GMS has been shown to be reliable between trained psychiatric interviewers, and agreement with clinical diagnosis is acceptable. It has also been shown to be sensitive to change over time (Copeland and Gurland 1978).

The length of the GMS makes it too unwieldy for use in more general surveys, or surveys mainly concerned with issues other than mental health. It is useful in epidemiological and psychiatric surveys focusing entirely or mainly on mental health. For further details, interested readers should consult the references given.

SHORT MENTAL-CONFUSION SCALES

Mental impairment is of such frequent occurrence among very elderly populations that a method of assessment during survey and evaluative research in this population group is now essential.

Mental-confusion tests generally have a fairly similar content and vary in length and complexity. There are several short 10-item tests in use worldwide. Each is culturally specific, although adaptations are minor (e.g. US scales ask about the name of the last President; UK scales ask about the name of the last Prime Minister or name of the Queen).

The Mental Status Questionnaire (MSQ)

The Mental Status Questionnaire is a concise measure of orientation and memory, drawn partly from standard mental-status examinations. It has been modified in the USA by Pfeiffer (1975) and reduced from 31 to 9 items. It has been widely used in community and clinical populations. It has been successfully used with older people living at home in the USA by Cornoni-Huntley et al. (1985) and has been judged to be a useful measure in institutional settings (Ebmeier et al. 1988). Wilson and Brass (1973) reported it could be easily administered to 90 per cent of geriatric-ward patients. They indicate that half the questions could be asked without the patient knowing s/he is being tested, and the other half can follow after brief explanation: 'How is your memory, I would like to test it?' They reported that it rarely provoked anxiety or embarrassment. It can be given without causing fatigue in the very ill.

There are many possible variations to this type of brief testing, e.g. Hodkinson's (1972) abbreviated Mental Test Score based on the longer version of that developed by Blessed et al. (1968).

Content

The 10 questions are:

Name of town
Address/name of place
Today's date (error of three days on either side of correct date allowed)
Month
Year
Age
Year of birth
Month of birth
Name of Prime Minister
Name of previous Prime Minister

Wilson and Brass (1973) found that item 1 could be excluded, as it contributed little to discrimination. The authors caution its use with deaf people and suggest writing down the questions, and acknowledged that it cannot be used with dysphasic patients.

Scoring

The number of correct cases are scored (correct=1; false=0).

Validity

Kahn *et al.* (1960b), on the basis of 1,066 patients in homes for the aged, nursing homes and state mental hospitals in New York City, reported that the MSQ was highly associated with psychiatrists' evaluations of the presence and degree of chronic brain syndrome. However, the authors simply reported percentage differences without significance values.

The association between the five items: town, place, age, month born, year born and the five test items: Prime Minister's name and current date, correlate fairly strongly; r:0.68 (Wilson and Brass 1973). Wilson and Brass concluded that the MSQ was a powerful measure for detecting and quantifying mental impairment.

Milne *et al.* (1972), in a longitudinal survey of mental health, compared results from the MSQ with the Mental Impairment Measurement, designed by Isaacs and Walkey (1964) and found the MSQ to be less sensitive than the latter.

Reliability

Kahn *et al.* (1960a; 1960b) reported reliability to be satisfactory. In a series of 55 cases, selected because their physical condition seemed likely to remain stable, the MSQ was administered four times at 3-week intervals: three-quarters of the scores changed by one or less (Wilson *et al.* 1973).

The Abbreviated Mental Test (AMT)

The Abbreviated Mental Test was developed by Hodkinson (1972) from the Modified Roth Hopkins Test (Blessed *et al.* 1968). The most discriminating items were incorporated. There was no evidence that patients' performance improved with practice.

Content

The test contains 10 items. These cover the following:

Age
Time (nearest hour)
Year
Name of place
Recognition of two persons

Birthday (date and month)
Date of World War I
Queen's name
Counting 20–1 backwards
5-minute recall: full street address

Scoring

Scores are totalled. Each correct item scores 1; maximum score: 10.

Validity

It has been further tested against the Crichton Royal Behaviour Rating Scale, and clinical diagnosis of dementia by Vardon and Blessed (1986), using 99 residents of homes for the elderly, with a mean age of 82.7. The authors reported that the AMT does reveal significant cognitive decline which is characteristic of dementias: over 80 per cent of residents allocated a clinical diagnosis of dementia scored 55 per cent or less correct answers on testing. It produced scores closely similar to those obtained on the Modified Roth Hopkins Test (Blessed *et al.* 1968). It has also been tested against a 37-item Roth-Hopkins test (AMT) by Thompson and Blessed (1987). These authors based their research on 52 mentally ill psychogeriatric day-care patients (mean age: 75). They reported that the 10-item test was better tolerated. The functionally ill scored consistently better than the organically ill. Correlations with longer mental-status scales were 0.91 to 0.96 which were comparable with those reported by Qureshi and Hodkinson (1974) for institutionalized patients (the latter reported correlations with longer mental-test scales of 0.87 to 0.96). Short versions of the AMT (which include 5 and 7 items) have been tested by Jitapunkel *et al.* (1991) with good results. It also has a higher sensitivity than the original.

Reliability

Although its authors have judged the test to be a brief, acceptable and reliable test of cognitive function, there is little published evidence regarding its reliability.

6
Measuring social networks and social support

Social-network analysis

Network models have been employed in numerous areas of sociology, psychology and anthropology. In research on health-care needs, lack of social support has been associated with increased mortality risk, delayed recovery from disease, poor morale and mental health (Lowenthal and Haven 1968; Berkman and Syme 1979; Bowling and Charlton 1987; Cohen et al. 1987; Lin et al. 1979; Maes et al. 1987; Seeman et al. 1987) although not everyone fits identical patterns, and research is also contradictory. Whatever the nature of the study, measuring social networks and support is fraught with difficulties, as most measures have not been fully tested for validity and reliability.

Social networks and social support are two different concepts. Network analysis was originally developed by sociologists and social anthropologists, although recent methodological advances have been due to the increasing involvement of social psychologists in this area (Mitchell and Trickett 1980). Sociologists believe that the characteristics of the network have some explanatory power of the social behaviour of the people involved (Mitchell 1969). The framework most applicable to the study of social support derives from the theory of social networks. This describes transactions among individuals. Each individual is a node in the network and each exchange a link. Networks are defined as the web of identified social relationships that surround an individual and the characteristics of those linkages. It is the set of people with whom one maintains contact and has some form of social bond. Social contacts and relationships are important ways for the individual to influence the environment and provide pathways through which the environment influences the individual (Saronson et al. 1977).

The importance of social networks, and their characteristics, lies in the extent to which they fulfil members' needs. Their functions can be summarized as 'that set of personal contacts through which the individual maintains his social identity, and receives emotional support, material aid, services, information and new social contacts' (Walker *et al.* 1977). House (1981) has suggested that social support involves emotional concern (liking, love); instrumental aid (services); information (about environment) and appraisal (information for self-evaluation). One approach to defining social support proceeds from a consideration of its source, such as who provides it; the functions it serves for people (e.g. material aid); and the intimacy characteristics of the relationship (e.g. whether it is a confiding relationship) (Tolsdorf 1976). Thus social support can be defined as the interactive process in which emotional, instrumental or financial aid is obtained from one's social network. Cobb (1976) defines social support as 'information leading the subject to believe that he is cared for and loved, esteemed, and a member of a network of mutual obligations'. Thus support exists only if it leads to certain beliefs in the recipient. Thoits (1982) has expanded this model to include instrumental aid. Despite several attempts to conceptualize social support, no agreement has yet been reached; attempts have been criticized as inadequate (Thoits 1982).

Several characteristics of networks appear relevant in terms of support. First, people must have connections with other people (network) in order to receive social support, but social connections do not guarantee access to social support. Other relevant dimensions are:

Size: the number of people maintaining social contact; this can include those who are only called on when needed

Geographic dispersion: networks vary from those confined by a household, to those in a single neighbourhood, and those that are more widely dispersed. Transport facilities may influence frequency of contact.

Density/integration: the extent to which network members are in each others' networks.

Composition and member homogeneity: friend, neighbour, children, sibling, other relatives; similarities between members (age, socioeconomic status, etc.).

Frequency of contact between members

Strength of ties: degree of intimacy; reciprocity; expectation of durability and availability, emotional intensity.

These structural characteristics of the network will influence:

Satisfactions with, and perceptions of the network and support/aid obtained.

Networks can thus be operationally defined in terms of size, geographic dispersion, strength of ties, density/integration, composition and member homogeneity (Craven and Wellman 1974; Mitchell 1969; Walker *et al.* 1977).

These structural characteristics are useful in calculating the number and distribution of relationships within a network and their degree of connection. The emerging patterns can then be studied in relation to the particular life situation of the individual. It can be hypothesized that different types of network structure have differing degrees of significance depending on the nature of need to be met.

'Dynamic features of the social network' refers to the positive or negative nature of network interactions. Analyses need to take account of the nature of human emotions involved. The size of the network and calculations of frequency of contact between members are of little value if these interactions are negative and stressful. It is also possible that the existence of a single confidant is of greater value in terms of meeting an individual's emotional needs than a larger number of more superficial friendships. The individual's subjective 'view' of the network takes into account the meaning of relationships and the strength of affectional ties. A different but related dimension is the concept of loneliness. This can be a consequence of perceived or actual poor emotional or social support. This concept and its measurement are discussed at the end of this chapter.

Methods of measurement

There is currently no assessment scale which comprehensively measures the main components of social network and support with acceptable levels of reliability and validity. Part of the problem stems from lack of agreement on conceptual bases, or even failure to consider these at all.

Many surveys have relied on single-item questions such as marital status, frequency of contact with others and existence of a confidant. Single-item measures have been found to be powerful predictors of health status and mortality but alone provide no insight into the dynamics of the network. It is important to match methodology to the empirical issue and correct disciplinary approach. Among the studies using only simple measures of social networks was the Alamada County Human Population Laboratory which provided the most convincing evidence of a link between social networks and mortality (Berkman and Syme 1979) but the precise nature of the relationship is unknown. If more studies used adequate measures, the links may prove to be stronger and the debate about links less controversial.

There is now a trend away from simple totalling of social contacts and single-item questions towards developing scales. Many earlier approaches simply assessed social network and support by questions on marital status and household composition (see review by Hirsch 1981). The implication from the early studies on social ties and mental and physical health is that social ties are important and merit further study. Studies relying on single-item questions and crude or simplistic measures cannot be used to derive substantive implications for practice. It is necessary to differentiate relationships according to their content, process and development. Failure to obtain these data precludes information on how social networks function as social support systems. Survey questions that do not separate social support from network structure do not permit identification of the social conditions under which help and support are provided. It cannot be assumed that having a daughter living nearby will necessarily lead to adequate support and help. Most attempts to measure quality of the network consist of questions asking respondents who they are close to, in contact with and if they see enough of the mentioned people. Such single items are inadequate as evaluations of the perceived quality of relationships (Adams 1967). Some assessment of satisfaction in relation to social support is essential, given that this has been found to be related to well-being, and its relationship to frequency of contact or perceived support is inconsistent in the literature (Fiore et al. 1986; Seeman and Berkman 1988).

Seeman and Berkman (1988) found that network characteristics do not appear to be so highly correlated with aspects of social support that they are interchangeable. Cohen et al. (1987), on the basis of their study of 155 elderly residents of midtown Manhattan single-room occupancy hotels, reported the results of a factor analysis showing that only 7 of the 19 network variables utilized had sufficient commonality to form a potential scale, suggesting that most variables are independent of each other. The authors criticize the use of scales without prior analysis of scale items and the development of scales without the use of parametric approaches such as factor analysis. As they point out, a possible problem with combining all network variables into one scale is the potential for premature treatment of network variables as unidimensional (i.e. representing one underlying construct). Combining variables which may be independent of each other into a simple scale may attenuate true variance and obscure differences which may be important. Much previous research has been limited to the use of bivariate statistical techniques, therefore making it impossible to control for overlap among variables or to determine the relative strength of variables. Measures of network need to be multi-faceted, taking into account structure and dynamic features of the network, as well as the individual's subjective perceptions of it.

Researchers often assume that measures of network size and frequency of social contacts are fairly 'objective' and stable in comparison with measures of the content and quality of relationships which are likely to be confounded by mental-health status (House and Kahn 1985). Donald and Ware (1982) reported one-year test-retest reliability coefficients of between 0.40 to 0.60 for reports of social contacts. One problem with network scales is that visits to relatives are so routine that they may be taken for granted and unreported as formal social visits (Stueve and Lein 1979). Spouses may also be so taken for granted as part of the network that they too are unreported in network scales (Bowling *et al.* 1988). Another problem with asking questions about social support is that feelings about the supportive nature of the network (affective component) are influenced by psychological well-being or depression as well as by network structure and functions. Thus people with adequate support may perceive it to be inadequate because they are feeling depressed. This problem has not been resolved. Subjective perceptions are, of course, important, but a measurement schedule should be able to distinguish between subjective and objective elements accurately. Perhaps additional interviews could be carried out with a member of the respondent's social network in order to establish the validity of the information provided by the respondent. Sokolovsky (1986) suggests an ethnographic approach to validate information given: participant observation, life histories, genealogies and informal interviews to probe the social support elements of social networks. An example is Francis's (1984) comparison of the Jewish elderly in Cleveland and England. Francis's methods were based on a comprehensive set of semi-structured questions centring around practical (transportation, shopping, money, etc.) and emotional (advice, visiting, etc.) services. Another example is Wentowski's (1982) study of an urban population in which he elicited examples of support as various events were reported.

In sum, there has been little attempt to test measures of social support for reliability and validity (Tardy 1985). Existing research generally suffers from methodological problems: imprecise definitions, failure to treat social support as a multidimensional concept, and various intervening variables confound studies. The main problem with most studies has been the inadequate conceptualization and operationalization of social support. It is common simply to itemize presence or absence of a spouse, confidant, household composition and social activities. Most researchers then total respondents' scores to questions about the structure of social networks and ignore the different dimensions of support. Conceptual definitions are more rarely offered, although sociologists are beginning to offer more developed conceptual statements: that the respondent believes s/he is cared for/loved/esteemed/valued and belongs to a network of significant others.

Available measures of social support

A selection of the available measures of social support have recently been optimistically reviewed by Payne and Graham-Jones (1987). These authors feel that existing measures can reasonably measure social support and fall down mainly on lack of testing for criterion validity. They fail to point out that far more evidence of all aspects of their reliability and validity is required before they can be used with confidence. On the other hand, it is encouraging that a start has been made in developing measures of this type. A number of these measures have also been briefly reviewed by Orth-Gomer and Unden (1987). They also reviewed a number of the shorter measures, consisting mainly of single-item questions with little reference to quality of, and satisfaction with, relationships, e.g. Berkman's Social Network Index (Berkman and Syme 1979); House's Social Relationships and Activities Scale (House *et al.* 1982); Lin's Social Support Scale (Lin *et al.* 1979) and Orth-Gomer and Johnson's Social Network Interaction Index (Orth-Gomer and Johnson 1987). Although these short-item measures appear to be inadequate in scope and depth, Berkman and Syme's, House's, and Orth-Gomer and Johnson's scale items do predict mortality. On the other hand, the items are insufficiently detailed to indicate precisely what dimensions of poor social-support structures are most important.

A review of 33 instruments purporting to measure social support by O'Reilly (1988) reported only modest agreement on conceptual definition and frequently the concepts were not defined or ill defined. In particular, definitional confusion between social network and social support was apparent. Variables used to operationalize these concepts reflected this conceptual confusion. For example, some of the measures he reviews define social support in terms of social-network characteristics (size, source and frequency of contact). O'Reilly was less optimistic about the value of existing measures and pointed out that more rigorous standards to establish validity and reliability were required.

Some of the more general measures of health status and quality of life include items on social support and activities; as these have been reviewed elsewhere in this volume, they will not be reviewed here (e.g. OARS; the Rand HIS batteries).

Inventory of Socially Supportive Behaviours (ISSB)

The ISSB is a measure designed by Barrera (1981) for use with a wide range of community populations. Social support was conceptualized as the diversity of natural helping behaviours that individuals actually receive, derived from the previous literature on social support. The authors felt that most existing scales concentrated on the structure of the network rather than what the members actually did, especially in view of noted discrepancies between actual amount of help provided and subjective perceptions of the amount of help (Liem and Liem 1978).

This scale is operationalized by 40 items generated from the literature to specify the amount of help received in the past month. The average time taken to complete the questionnaire is about ten minutes.

Content

The ISSB measures four types of support: emotional, instrumental, information appraisal and socializing. The index asks respondents to state how people have helped them in the last month and to respond on a five-point Likert-type scale to each of the 40 items as 'not at all', 'once or twice', 'about once a week', 'several times a week' or 'about every day'. It measures the receipt of support, but not the source. Examples of items which ask if anyone has given them support include:

Expressed interest and concern in your well-being.
Listened to you talk about your private feelings.
Was right there with you (physically) in a stressful situation.

Items on instrumental appraisal support:
Provided you with a place where you could get away for a while.
Loaned you over $25.
Provided you with some transportation.

Informational appraisal support:
Gave you some information on how to do something.
Gave you feedback on how you were doing without saying it was good or bad.
Helped you understand why you didn't do something well.

Socializing:
Talked to you about some interest of yours.
Did some activity together to help you get your mind off things.

There is a problem with all these statements in that they may or may not relate to real events in people's immediate lives, and some items may measure resources available to the supporter rather than support to the respondents (e.g. items on financial and car loans).

Scoring

The five-point ratings of each item are summed to produce a total score, with higher scores indicating greater support. The author also suggests calculating an average frequency score as this permits a global score to be produced when there is some missing data for items.

A weakness with scales of this type is that, without a distinction between available and enacted support, the scale may simply be measuring the number, type and severity of problems recently experienced by the respondent.

Validity

The validity of the ISSB was tested by correlating results, based on 43 students, with a measure of family relations (Family Environment Scale); the correlation, although significant, was not high: 0.35. The author speculated that this was because the two scales were measuring different dimensions of support. Construct validity was assumed by correlations of the index with a measure of life events: 0.38 to 0.41 (Barrera 1981; Sandler and Barrera 1984). Notes available from the author on the scale summarize the correlations between ISSB and measures of distress from ten published studies. The correlations range from 0.01 to 0.50, although most were fairly weak.

Two published studies have addressed the dimensionality of the ISSB empirically; each involved exploratory factor analysis and showed considerable agreement (Barrera and Ainlay 1983; Stokes and Wilson 1984). An unpublished study by Caldwell and Reinhart is also consistent with these analyses and labels the clusters as Guidance, Emotional Support and Tangible Support.

Reliability

The test-retest reliability correlation coefficient, based on 71 students tested over two days, was 0.88; test-retest reliability coefficients, again using students, over a one-month period were 0.80 and 0.63 (Barrera 1981; Barrera and Ainlay 1983; Valdenegro and Barrera 1983). Internal-consistency reliability coefficients of 0.92 and 0.94 were reported for the first and second administrations of the scale (Barrera 1981). Notes on the ISSB are available from the author at Arizona State University; these report that tests from five studies show the internal consistency coefficients of the scale to be above 0.90.

In sum, there are problems with interpretation of the scale. Also, although preliminary results for reliability testing appear good, far more work on both the reliability and validity of the scale is needed before it can be recommended.

Arizona Social Support Interview Schedule (ASSIS)

The ISSB (above) was not designed to provide information on people who supplied resources, nor respondents' subjective appraisals of the adequacy of support. Barrera subsequently designed the Arizona Social Support Interview Schedule (ASSIS) to address this gap. The ASSIS was developed by Barrera (1980; 1981) as an instrument to measure several aspects of support, including procedures for identifying support-network membership and subjects' satisfaction with and need for support. His conceptual definition, based on previous literature, of social network relates to people who provide the functions defined as support. The scale is based on self-report and takes 15–20 minutes to complete.

Content

The scale is operationalized by asking subjects to identify individuals who provide support in the following areas: private feelings, material aid, advice, positive feedback, physical assistance and social participation. In each area, subjects are asked about such support from the named individuals in the past month, and whether the support was sufficient; ratings of satisfaction are made on a three-point scale. Examples of items are:

Private feelings

1 If you wanted to talk to someone about things that are very personal and private, who would you talk to? Give me the first names, initials, or nicknames of the people that you would talk to about things that are very personal and private.
Probe: is there anyone else that you can think of?

2 During the last month, which of these people did you actually talk to about things that were personal and private?
Probe: Ask specifically about people who were listed in response to 1 but not listed in response to 2.

3 During the last month, would you have liked:
   1 A lot more opportunities to talk to people about your personal and private feelings?
   2 A few more opportunities?
   3 Or was this about right?

4 During the past month, how much do you think you needed people to talk about things that were very personal and private?
   1 Not at all.
   2 A little bit.
   3 Quite a bit.

Social participation

1 Who are the people you get together with to have fun or relax? These could be new names or ones you listed before.
Probe: anyone else?

2 During the past month, which of these people did you actually get together with to have fun or relax?
Probe: ask about people who were named in 1 but not 2.

3 During the past month, would you have liked:
1 A lot more opportunities to get together with people for fun and relaxation?
2 A few more?
3 Or was it about right?

How much do you think you needed to get together with other people for fun and relaxation during the past month?
1 Not at all?
2 A little bit?
3 Quite a bit?

The interview schedule also includes questions concerning negative interactions, on the basis of the psychiatric literature linking these to mental disturbance (identification of people with whom they have had conflicts in the past month). Finally, subjects are asked about the age, sex and ethnicity of people named.

Scoring

The data obtained allow the calculation of specified scores from the relevant items of total available and total utilized network size, conflict network size, unconflicted network size, amount of support satisfaction and support need. The author reported that the support-satisfaction measure suffers from an extremely skewed distribution in the direction of high satisfaction scores (Barrera 1981). Notes which identify the item scores which should be used in calculations are available from the author at Arizona State University.

Validity

The predictive validity was tested on a sample of 86 pregnant adolescents. It was reported by Barrera (1981) that conflicted network size correlated significantly with depression and anxiety, satisfaction correlated with depression and anxiety, and expressed need correlated significantly with depression and anxiety and somatization (0.23–0.51).

The reported relationship between life events and social support was taken as evidence for the index's construct validity (0.25 to 0.38), although these correlations are at best modest. The ASSIS was administered along with the ISSB. The ISSB showed a modest but significant correlation with total network size (0.32), but was not significantly correlated with satisfaction or need on the ASSIS.

Reliability

The instrument has been tested for test-retest reliability, and results appear moderately satisfactory to good. It was tested on 45 students and total network size produced a correlation coefficient of 0.88 over three days, and studies with a further group of students produced a test-retest correlation over one month of 0.70 (Barrera 1980; Valdenegro and Barrera 1983). Test-retest correlations were 0.54 for size of conflicted network, 0.69 for satisfaction and 0.80 for support need. There was also modest support for predictive and construct validity (Barrera 1981).

Internal consistency correlations for support satisfaction and support need were low to moderate: 0.33 and 0.52 respectively.

A study by Barrera *et al.* (1985) of 36 mental-health out-patients who agreed to supply the name of one network member showed significant kappa coefficients between subjects' and informants' reports of support. Of the 31 cases of non-agreement of ASSIS items, 24 were due to informants' stating that they had provided aid when subjects indicated that they had not; and seven were due to subjects reporting that aid was provided and informants did not.

Further testing for both reliability and validity is required. At best the validity of the scale is modest.

Perceived Social Support from Family and Friends

This was devised by Procidano and Heller (1983) as a measure of perceived social support. It was designed to assess the functions of social networks specified by Caplan (1974): 'the extent to which an individual perceives that his/her needs for support, information, and feedback are fulfilled by friends... and by family'. Thoits (1982) has criticized this definition as inadequate on the grounds that it includes the very term to be defined (support). The scale measures available and received support, especially emotional support. It takes about eight minutes to complete.

Content

It comprises two 20-item self-report measures, derived, after testing with students, from an initial pool of 84 items. One 20-item measure is for perceptions of family support and one 20-item measure is for perceptions of support from/given by friends. Responses require a simple 'yes', 'no', or 'don't know'. Examples are:

Family
I rely on my family for emotional support;
My family is sensitive to my personal needs;
My family gives me the moral support I need.

Friends
My friends enjoy hearing about what I think;
I have a deep, sharing relationship with a number of friends;
I feel that I'm on the fringe of my circle of friends.

A few items refer to support given:
My friends come to me for emotional support;
Certain members of my family come to me when they have problems or need advice.

Scoring

Positive item responses are totalled and presented separately for family and friends. An overall score can also be calculated.

Validity

The authors reported that the scale correlated with measures of psycho-pathology and distress (0.85–0.98) therefore demonstrating predictive and construct validity. The sensitivity of scale is unknown.

Reliability

In relation to internal consistency, tests with 222 students produced correlation coefficients of 0.88 and 0.90 respectively for the items relating to family and those relating to friends. Test–retest reliability, using 222 students, was 0.83 over a one-month period.

Although the scale has good internal reliability, test–retest reliability and predictive validity, far more testing is required.

Social Support Questionnaire

This questionnaire was developed by Sarason *et al.* (1983) to measure the availability of, and satisfaction with, social support. The conceptual definition of support was derived from Bowlby's theory of attachment and is based on the existence or availability of people who can be relied upon, who care about, love and value the recipient.

In the construction of the scale, which is based on self-report, 61 items were written to sample the situations in which social support might be important to people. They were administered to 602 students who were asked to list people who provided them with such support. Items that showed low correlations with other items were deleted. Scoring methods were also piloted. The scoring method selected was the simplest – a count of supportive persons. The availability index selected was the number of persons listed divided by the number of items.

Most of the items are concerned with emotional support, so this scale is appropriate for measurement of emotional support only. The scale takes an average of fifteen minutes to complete.

Content

The instrument comprises 27 items which ask the subjects (a) to list all the people to whom they can turn in specific situations and (b) to indicate their satisfaction with each of these identified supports on a scale ranging from very satisfied to very dissatisfied. Examples are:

Whom can you really count on to listen to you when you need to talk?
Whom could you really count on to help you out in a crisis situation, even though
   they would have to go out of their way to do so?
With whom can you totally be yourself?
Whom can you really count on to be dependable when you need help?
Who do you feel really appreciates you as a person?
Whom can you count on to console you when you are very upset?

Scoring

Each item is scored (number of persons listed); the satisfaction score ranges from 1 to 6 (very satisfied to not very satisfied). Two scores are computed by dividing the sum of each of the two scores (number of people; overall satisfaction) by the 27 items: average (per item) number of people, and average level of satisfaction with support.

Validity

Attempts were made by the authors to test the construct validity of the scale. Sarason *et al.* (1983) reported a study of 227 students who were administered the scale along with personality scales (extraversion and neuroticism). The correlations with the Social Support Questionnaire were weak to moderate: −0.02 and −0.43 for availability and satisfaction with support. Another study they reported with 295 students showed an association between positive life events and number of social supports. And a study with 440 students showed that people with more social supports had more positive self-concepts.

Predictive validity was judged to be satisfactory on the basis of correlations with depression (the correlations for 100 men and 127 women for each dimension were from −0.22 to −0.43. The sensitivity of the scale is largely unknown.

Separate factor analyses were performed by the authors for each of the two scores. Each analysis showed a very strong first (unrotated) factor. The first factor accounted for 82 per cent of the common variance for the availability score, and 72 per cent for the satisfaction with support score. All factor loadings exceeded 0.60 and 0.30 for each score respectively. There appeared to be good evidence that one strong factor underlies each score and that they represent different dimensions of the concept.

Reliability

Test-retest reliability over a four-week period, using 602 students, was 0.90 for the availability of support items, and 0.83 for satisfaction with support, using 105 students. The alpha coefficients for internal reliability were 0.97 for availability and 0.94 for satisfaction with support, using 602 university students. Inter-item correlations ranged from 0.37 to −0.71 for availability, and from 0.21 to −0.74 for satisfaction with support. A second study of 227 students showed a correlation between the availability and satisfaction with support scores of 0.31 for men and 0.21 for women (Sarason et al. 1983).

In sum, it is a viable measure of support, with good results for internal reliability; construct validity has been demonstrated and predictive validity modest. Again, more work on its validity and reliability is required.

Interview Schedule for Social Interaction (ISSI)

This index was developed by Henderson et al. (1980). The conceptual definition of support was based on the theory that social relations are based on attachment, social integration, nurturance, reassurance of personal worth, sense of reliability, help and guidance. The scale was developed over a year in pilot studies of 130 people in health centres, out-patient departments in a club for the elderly, and in a general population sample in Canberra. It was reported to be acceptable to both healthy and psychiatrically disturbed respondents.

The scale takes approximately 30 minutes to complete, although reports of 60 minutes have also been published.

Content

The scale comprises 52 questions asking about the availability and adequacy of people in specific roles: attachment, provided by close affectional relationships; social integration, provided by membership of a network of persons having shared interests and values; the opportunity for nurturing others; reassurance of personal worth; a sense of reliable alliance; and obtaining help and guidance from informal advisers in times of difficulty. It does not adequately measure the availability and adequacy of attachment and social integration.

A question about the availability of provision is immediately followed by a question on adequacy. Examples are:

How many friends do you have whom you could visit at any time, without waiting for an invitation? You could arrive without being expected and still be sure you would be welcome.

Would you like to have more or fewer friends like this, or is it about right for you?

Three items ask about negative interactions:

How many people whom you have to see regularly do you dislike?

Scoring

The four principal indices yield four scores: availability of attachment, perceived adequacy of attachment, availability of social integration and perceived adequacy of social integration. The following indices are created:

AVAT: the availability of affectionally close relationships (attachments)
ADAT: the perceived adequacy of what comprises these close relationships, expressed as a percentage of what is available
NONAT: those who lack close relationships, might not be unhappy with their situation. The NONDAT index is a measure of such satisfaction despite the absence of attachment.
ATTROWN: the number of attachment persons with whom the respondents has been having rows in the last month.
AVSI: the availability of more diffuse relationships, as with friends, work associates and acquaintances (social integration).
ADSI: the perceived adequacy of these more diffuse relationships.

Validity

The authors judged the scale to have face validity on the basis of its content. They suggested that the items effectively tap the constructs of availability and adequacy of attachment in adulthood and social integration.

Henderson *et al.* (1980) established the construct validity of the scale by analysing its four dimensions in relation to personality assessments (neuroticism and introversion–extraversion as measured by the Eysenck Personality Inventory). The sample comprised 225 members of the general population. Inverse relationships with availability and satisfaction measures and neuroticism were reported (–0.18 to –0.31). Results were less consistent with extraversion. The authors argued that one would predict that a neurotic person would have problems in forming and maintaining social relationships and would consequently be dissatisfied with those relationships.

Predictive validity was reported by the authors on the basis of a study of neurosis based on 751 residents of Canberra, Australia. The measure was associated with Zung's Self Rating Depression Scale and Goldberg's General Health Questionnaire (–0.15 to –0.96) (Henderson 1981). The study, which was based on baseline data collection from 756 residents in Canberra, with three follow-up interviews with a sub-sample over twelve months, reported that deficiencies in social relationships had an effect on the early development of neurotic symptoms. As both availability and adequacy items correlated significantly and negatively with psychiatric disorder and depression, predictive validity was judged to be satisfactory. The scale was also able to discriminate between new migrants to Canberra and those who had been living there for seven months or more. The strength of this study was that it was carried out on a representative sample of the population and was prospective, not cross-sectional; thus the measures of social ties were less likely to be contaminated by already established neurotic symptoms. The correlations between respondents' ISSI scores and those of someone who was nominated as well informed about their social relationships were weak to moderate, although significant, ranging between 0.26 and 0.59 for the items. This may be an indicator of the difference between actual and perceived support.

Reliability

Test-retest reliability scores for the scale indices over an 18-day period using 51 people from the general population ranged from 0.71 to 0.76; using 756 adults from a general population over an 18-day period, scores ranged from 0.66 to 0.85, and over a 12-month period ranged from 0.66 to 0.85. The problem with this long time period is that support structures might have changed and thus a lower correlation may reflect this rather than the reliability of the measure. Internal consistency reliability coefficients range from 0.67 to 0.81 for the indices.

In sum, although this is a promising scale, again more testing is required.

The Social Network Scale (SNS)

The Social Network Scale was adapted by Stokes (1983), based on Hirsch's (1980) work. This work was based on just 20 recent young widows and 14 older women recently re-entering college studies. Stokes (1983) based the Social Network Scale on four dimensions of network that he judged to be important: network size, number of people the respondent feels close to, number of relatives in the network and network density.

A supplement to the SNS is an eight-item scale which asks subjects to rate their total social networks, and their networks of friends, on four dimensions: general satisfaction with the network, amount of desired change in the network, satisfaction with assistance in daily activities, and satisfaction with emotional support. The eight ratings are summed to provide a measure of satisfaction.

Content

Hirsch's (1980) conceptual definition of support was based on interaction that affects coping ability: guidance, social reinforcement, aid, socializing, and emotional support. The social support dimension of the scale was operationalized by asking respondents to specify the amount of interaction with network members in five areas of supportive activity, and their degree of satisfaction with the interaction.

The social network dimension of the scale conceptualized social network as a natural support system, based on significant others. This is operationalized by asking subjects to list in a matrix 'the initials of up to 20 people who are significant in your life and with whom you have contact at least once a month'. Subjects then put an X in those boxes of the matrix that connect people who are significant in each other's lives and who have contact with each other at least once a month. Subjects also indicate which persons in their lists are relatives, and which persons they can 'confide in or turn to for help in an emergency'. This is probably more important in terms of providing effective, satisfying support than network size (Brown et al. 1975; Conner et al. 1979; Stokes 1983). This yields information on:

1. The size of the network, taking the definition of network as people who are significant in the respondent's life and with whom the respondent interacts regularly.
2. The number of people in the network whom the respondent feels close to – how many one can confide in or turn to for help in an emergency.
3. The number of relatives in the network.
4. Network density (i.e. the degree to which network members are themselves interconnected).

Scoring

Scoring consists of totalling the number of network members, relatives and confidantes. Scoring could also identify the overlap between these categories (e.g. between relatives and confidantes).

A larger number of variables can be computed and scored from the grid:

(i)   Network size: number of people listed
(ii)   Relatives: number of relatives listed
(iii)   Friends: number of people listed who are not relatives
(iv)   Confidantes: number of people subjects said they could confide in or turn to for help in an emergency
(v)   Relative confidantes: number of confidantes who are relatives
(vi)   Friend confidantes: number of confidantes who are not relatives
(vii)   Percentage relatives: proportion of the network who are relatives (relatives/size)
(viii) Percentage confidantes: proportion of the network members who are confidantes (confidantes/size)
(ix)   Percentage relative confidantes: proportion of confidantes who are relatives (relative confidantes/confidantes)
(x)   Density: the proportion of the total possible number of relationships which actually exist among members of a social network, excluding the respondent
(xi)   Relative density: density of the relatives in the social network list
(xii)   Friend density: density of the friends in the social network list
(xiii) Relative–friend density: number of relationships between relatives and friends as a proportion of the total possible number of such relationships.

Validity and reliability

Although the scale has been judged to have face validity, it has not been tested fully for reliability and validity. It is also limited in scope; Stokes has himself supplemented the use of the SNS with other scales measuring the frequency of receipt of support (e.g. the Inventory of Socially Supportive Behaviours (Stokes, 1985)). Stokes (1983), on the basis of administering the SNS to 82 students, submitted these dimensions to a principal components analysis and four factors emerged which accounted for over 80 per cent of the variance in the original matrix: size, with emphasis on the number of friends in the network; presence of confidantes; dominance of relatives in the network; and density. The procedure had the advantage of providing these measures which were uncorrelated with one another.

It is not clear what the basis for limiting social network members to twenty is. Also, a flaw with calculating the percentage of relatives, confidantes or friends in the network is that this does not take account of size in the presentation: for example, a network composed of 50 per cent relatives could be a network of just two members, one of whom is a relative, or it could be a network size of twenty, ten of whom are relatives. This does not appear to be a satisfactory basis for making comparisons between respondents.

Other main problems with this scale are that it does not have an index of geographical proximity, or frequency of contact, of network members, and it does not distinguish between types of relatives (e.g. sons and daughters are not distinguishable) or the nature of the contact (supportive, instrumental, etc). Moreover, the author's own experience with the scale is that respondents tend to omit their spouses from the network scale – their significance and contact being taken for granted (Bowling et al 1988).

The social support part of the scale has been little tested but was judged to have face reliability; the correlation between subject and interviewer ratings of satisfaction and support was 0.53 and was judged to be reliable. Inter-item correlations, testing for reliability, ranged from 0.22 to 0.51 (Hirsch 1980).

The sensitivity of the scale is unknown and more evidence of its reliability and validity is required. Generally, it will require supplementation with other items.

The Family Relationship Index (FRI)

The Family Relationship Index attempts to measure support from within the family. It has no clear conceptual basis. It was developed by Moos and Moos (1981) and Billings and Moos (1982). It was derived from a 90-item true–false response choice instrument, with 10 sub-scales, called the Family Environment Scale also developed by the authors. The scale was initially developed with a number of normal and distressed families in different ethnic groups. Over a thousand families were involved.

Content

The FRI subscale is composed of three sections (Moos and Moos 1981), taken from the Family Environment Scale. The three sections relate to 'cohesion', 'expressiveness' and 'conflict'. The 'cohesion' section assesses the amount of commitment, assistance and sustenance family members contribute to each other; 'expressiveness' assesses the extent to which family members are encouraged to express their feelings directly; and 'conflict' assesses the extent to which family members express aggression, conflict or anger. The three sections, with examples of item response choices, are:

Cohesion – the degree to which family members are helpful and supportive of each other (e.g. 'There is a feeling of togetherness in our family.');

Expressiveness – the extent to which family members are encouraged to act openly and to express their feelings directly (e.g. 'We tell each other about our personal problems.');

Conflict – the extent to which the open expression of anger and aggression and generally conflictual interactions are characteristic of the family (e.g. 'We fight a lot in our family.').

Scoring

The standardized scores of each subscale are averaged to produce a composite score. A manual is available (Moos and Moos 1981).

Validity

Although there is no reference to the predictive validity of the full scale in the manual, the Family Relationship subscale was reported to have predictive validity by Billings and Moos (1982) in their longitudinal study of social support and functioning among 113 patients who had been treated for alcoholism. However, not all correlations achieved statistical significance: the significant correlations reported were those for depression and level and source of reported support (0.19 to 0.74); it is known that people who are depressed tend to perceive their level of support to be lower. There has been little further testing of the scale. The validity and sensitivity of the full scale and the subscale are largely unknown.

Reliability

The FRI was reported by Billings and Moos (1981) and Holahan and Moos (1981) to have a high internal consistency (0.89) and to be related to other measures of social support.

Test-retest reliabilities for the full Family Environment Scale's 10 subscales at intervals of 8 weeks, 4 months and 12 months ranged between 0.52 and 0.89 (Moos and Moos 1981; Caldwell 1985).

In sum, although tests for reliability appear to be good, the validity of the scale is more questionable, and again the need for further testing is evident. Caldwell (1985), in his critique of the scale, states that the full instrument is useful if used with 'caution', given, in particular, the lack of evidence regarding its psychometric properties.

The Social Support Appraisals Scale (SS-A) and the Social Support Behaviours Scale (SS-B)

The Social Support Appraisals Scale was developed by Vaux *et al.* (1986a; 1986b). The concept of social support employed was based on Cobb's (1976) definition of social support and was designed to tap the extent to which individuals believe that they are loved by, esteemed by and involved with family, friends and others. One main advantage is the brevity of the scale.

Content: SS-A

The SS-A is a 23-item scale consisting of a list of statements about relationships with family and friends. Eight items relate to family relationships, seven to relationships with friends and eight to 'others' in a general way. Respondents have four response choices: 'strongly agree', 'agree', 'disagree' or 'strongly disagree'. There is no middle value. Examples are:

My friends respect me
My family cares for me very much
I am not important to others
I am well liked
I feel a strong bond with my friends
If I died tomorrow very few people would miss me
I feel close to members of my family
My friends and I have done a lot for one another
(Strongly agree/agree/disagree/strongly disagree)

Scoring

Three scores can be computed: SS-A, which is the sum of all 23 items; SS-A (family) which is the sum of the eight family items; and SS-A (friends) which is the sum of the seven friends items. The limitation of the scale is that it provides no information about the numbers of people involved in providing supportive behaviour, nor of who they are (e.g. spouse, sister, son, etc.).

Validity

Convergent and divergent validity was tested in relation to five samples of students and five community samples (the total number of respondents was around a thousand). It was tested against other measures of social support (the Perceived Social Support Scale; the Family Relations Index; the Social Support Questionnaire and two other less well-known scales; and three single-item questions on satisfaction with friends). The authors also employed two further scales developed by themselves. One of these was the Social Support Resources Scale. This was designed to tap many aspects of the individual's social support network. Respondents are asked to list up to ten people who provide them with five types of support: emotional support, practical assistance, financial assistance, socializing and advice/guidance. Respondents provide satisfaction ratings for the five types of assessed support. Respondents are asked further questions about the characteristics of the people identified and the nature of the relationship (e.g. spouse, friend). Mean scores are computed for each variable. The final scale tested against the SS-A was the Social Support Behaviours Scale, also developed by the authors (see below). The authors also tested the SS-A against six personality and depression inventories, including the Affect-Balance Scale, and the UCLA Revised Loneliness Scale (see pages 146 and 157).

The authors provided evidence of convergent validity with a variety of the support measures. The vast number of correlation coefficients presented by the authors is too extensive to reproduce here. However, none of the correlations with other support or personality measures were very strong (ranging from 0.03 to −0.51, with one correlation coefficient achieving −0.72). This is not surprising given the very different theoretical concepts underlying the different scales.

Reliability

There is no published evidence of reliability.

In sum, the validity of this part of the scale remains questionable, and evidence of reliability is also required.

Content: SS-B

The Social Support Behaviours Scale, was developed by Vaux et al. (1987) to tap five modes of supportive behaviour. It is similar to Barrera et al.'s ISSB (see page 125) but does not suffer from the limitation of asking solely about actual rather than potential support (which may simply reflect number of problems). This lists 45 specific supportive behaviours, tapping the five modes of support listed in their Social Support Resources scale: emotional support, socializing, practical assistance, financial assistance and advice/guidance. Respondents indicate how likely their family and friends would be to engage in each of the behaviours in time of need. Examples are:

Would suggest doing something, just to take my mind off my problems.
Would visit with me, or invite me over.
Would give me a ride if I needed one.
Would have lunch or dinner with me.
Would loan me a car if I needed one.
Would go to a movie or concert with me.

(No one would do this/someone might do this/some family member/friends would probably do this/some family member/friend would certainly do this/most family members/friends would certainly do this.)

A problem with these types of scales is that they assume social values, i.e. that respondents all equally value 'a movie or concert', and that other people are in a financial position to, for example, 'loan a car'.

Scoring

The choice of five responses for each type of behaviour itemized ranges from 'no one would do this' to 'most family members/friends would certainly do this' (see above). Items are scored 0 (no one) to 5 (certainly) and summed.

Validity

The predictive validity of the SS–B has been demonstrated in relation to psychological distress and it correlates moderately with other support measures (including SS–A, see overleaf) (Vaux and Wood 1985; Vaux et al. 1986a; 1986b).

In addition, five methods were used to test the validity of the SS–B as a measure of support: the classification of items by judges; an analogue (role-playing) simulation of samples deficient in each mode of support; tests against a related measure of supportive behaviour (ISSB); an examination of levels of each type of support provided for different problems and confirmatory factory analysis (Vaux et al. 1987).

The classification of items according to their content by judges (students) provided some evidence of the content validity of the SS–B. The percentage of items correctly classified by judges ranged from 13 to 100 per cent; in most cases it was over 60 per cent. The unique role-playing exercise with students showed deficits in available support corresponding to their enacted role, providing evidence of sub-scale sensitivity. However, the correlations were weak with the ISSB. This may be because the two measures are based on different concepts of social support – available and enacted respectively. The factor analysis demonstrated that the pattern of item convergence and divergence was highly consistent with predictions and confirmed that the SS–B taps the five modes of support conceptualized very well.

Reliability

Excellent internal consistency was obtained for the SS–B Scale items (the lowest alpha was 0.82).

In sum, the SS–A and SS–B scales are promising but have been little tested for reliability and validity.

Interpersonal Support Evaluation List (ISEL)

The Interpersonal Support Evaluation List was developed by Cohen *et al.* (1985), on the basis of the theoretical assumption that the buffering effect of social support is cognitively mediated. The testing of this theoretical assumption required an instrument which aimed to measure the perceived availability of support. The items were developed on theoretical grounds to cover the domain of social support that could facilitate coping with stress. It was designed to assess perceived availability of support in four distinct areas: material aid (tangible subscale); someone to talk to about one's problems (appraisal subscale); comparisons of self with others (self-esteem subscale); people to share activities with (belonging subscale).

Content

The ISEL consists of a list of 40 (48 in the version for students) statements about the perceived availability of potential social resources. The items are balanced: half the statements comprising the scale contain positive items about social relationships, and half contain negative items.

Respondents are asked to indicate whether each statement is 'probably true' or 'probably false'. Examples of the items are:

There is at least one person I know whose advice I really trust.
There are very few people I trust to help solve my problems.
If I decide on a Friday afternoon that I would like to go to a movie that evening, I could find someone to go with me.
Most people I know don't enjoy the same things that I do.
If I were sick and needed someone to drive me to the doctor, I would have trouble finding someone.
If I had to mail an important letter at the post office by 5.00 and couldn't make it, there is someone who could do it for me.
In general people don't have much confidence in me.
Most people I know think highly of me.

Scoring

The ISEL is scored by counting the number of responses indicating support. There is no information on the validity of this method.

Validity

Cohen *et al*. (1985) reviewed the evidence on the reliability and validity of the scale, most of which was previously unpublished. The scale was tested on over 500 students in Oregon; over 100 students at Carnegie-Mellon University; almost 100 students at Delaware University; over 100 students at Guelph University; and over 100 students at Arizona State University. Four studies were also carried out on the version of the scale for the general population using student samples at the University of California, Carnegie-Mellon University and the University of Oregon (total: over 200 students), and a general population sample participating in the Oregon Smoking Cessation Program (over 60 adults).

The ISEL student scale was found to correlate moderately with other social-support scales: 0.46 with Barrera's ISSB; 0.30 with the total score of the Moos Family Environment Scale; 0.39 with reported network size; 0.46 with number of close friends reported; and 0.42 with number of close relatives reported. The scale for the general population correlated 0.31 with a scale measuring the quality of relationships with partner/ spouse. It was expected that the scale would be associated with self-esteem, as this is influenced by feedback from others; the correlation with the Rosenberg Self-Esteem Scale (see p. 167) was 0.74. The scale was reported to be significantly associated with depression; social anxiety was controlled to eliminate the possibility that the social support concept was not merely a proxy measure of personality (e.g. social anxiety or social skills). Longitudinal analyses of the groups in the studies showed that the scale was able to predict changes in depressive symptomatology. The latter association indicated that the scale is not simply measuring symptomatology. There was a small but significant association with physical symptomatology and changes in these symptoms. The scale was reported to be a good predictor of smoking cessation and was associated with measures of stress in the direction suggestive of the buffering effects of social support. The authors argue that these data suggest the importance of appraisal support as a protector against the pathogenic effects of stressful life events.

Reliability

Adequate internal and test-retest reliability was reported by the authors.

With the scale for students, the internal-reliability alpha coefficient was 0.86, ranging from 0.60 to 0.92 for each subscale. The alpha coefficients for the general population scale ranged from 0.88 to 0.90. The subscale correlations ranged from 0.62 to 0.82.

The student scales were tested for test-retest reliability at four-week intervals with reported correlations of 0.87 for the total scale, and correlations of 0.71 – 0.87 for the subscales. The general population scale was administered twice with a two-day interval; the reported correlation for the total scale was 0.87, and the subscale correlations ranged from 0.67 to 0.84. The six-week test-retest correlations from the smoking-cessation group sample were 0.70 overall, and 0.63 – 0.69 for the subscales. The six-month test-retest correlations for this group were 0.74 for the total scale, and 0.49 – 0.68 for the subscales. In sum, although this is a scale which has only recently been developed, and further testing is required, it does cover a wide range of supportive relationships and results of testing for reliability and validity are fairly good. One limitation is that the scale does appear to be orientated towards a young or active population group and so may not be suitable for use with frail elderly people (e.g. questions on advice over job changes, sexual problems and availability of people to give lifts to the airport, etc.).

Loneliness

A further concept requires introduction under the heading of social networks and support: that of loneliness. Loneliness can be defined as an unwelcome feeling of lack or loss of companionship. Weiss (1973) distinguished between situational and personality theories of loneliness. The former emphasize environmental factors as causes of loneliness – e.g. death of a spouse, moving to a new city. Evidence relating to the size and quality of social networks and associations with loneliness is unclear. Apart from a number of psychological studies which are of questionable generalizability as they tend to use student volunteers as subjects, the quality of data on loneliness in relation to the quality of social networks are poor. Most surveys have either been based on small sample sizes or have used crude measures of social network or loneliness (Jones et al. 1985; Bowling et al. 1989).

Although a large number of scales for the assessment of loneliness have been devised, few have been published. The existing scales have been reviewed by Russell (1982). The most widely used scale is the UCLA Loneliness Scale, and this is reviewed below.

The Revised University of California at Los Angeles (UCLA) Loneliness Scale

The UCLA Loneliness Scale is the most well-known measure of loneliness. It was developed, and later revised, by Russell *et al.* (1978; 1980). The authors aimed to identify common themes that characterized the experience of loneliness for a broad spectrum of individuals. The UCLA Loneliness Scale was intended to be global.

The scale began with 25 items taken from another measure. The response items, also borrowed, asked individuals to rate how frequently they felt the way described, from 'never' to 'often' on a four-point scale. The scale was tested on clinic volunteers and students. The final loneliness scale consisted of 20 items; selected items all had item–total correlations above 0.50.

One problem with the original version of the scale was that all the items on the measure were worded in the same (lonely) direction. The implication is that tendencies to respond in a certain way could systematically influence loneliness scores. A second potential problem was social-desirability bias, given the possible stigma associated with admissions of loneliness. Thus Russell *et al.* (1980) revised the scale to take account of these problems, and a set of positively worded loneliness items were included (e.g. 'There are people I feel close to.' and 'I have a lot in common with the people around me.'). The revised version was tested on 162 students. Testing involved using the original scale and 19 new items, written by the authors, and anxiety and depression measures. The ten positively and ten negatively worded items with the highest correlations with a set of items about whether they were lonely were included in the scale. All of the item–criterion correlations were above 0.40.

Content

The scale consists of 20 statements, half of which are descriptive of feelings of loneliness and half descriptive of non-loneliness or satisfaction with relationships. Examples of items are:

I lack companionship.
It is difficult for me to make friends.
There is no one I can turn to.
I feel part of a group of friends.
There are people I feel close to.

Respondents indicate how often each statement applies to them. There are four choices for replies: never (1), rarely (2), sometimes (3) and often (4).

Scoring

The total score of the scale is the sum of all 20 items. Some need to be reversed before scoring (i.e. 1=4, 2=3, 3=2, 4=1); these are asterisked on the scale.

Validity

Validity was initially assessed by correlations of the scale with a single-item self-rating of loneliness measure (0.79); a comparison of the scores of two samples of participants (the mean of the clinic sample was 60.1, significantly different from the student group's mean of 39.1); and the loneliness scores were also strongly associated with depression, anxiety, dissatisfaction, unhappiness and shyness. High correlations with other measures of loneliness have been reported (ranging from 0.72 and 0.74). These have been reviewed by Russell (1982). The main limitation of this research is that it has been largely confined to samples of students, raising questions about the validity of the scale in assessing loneliness for other populations. Although there is a need for further testing of the scale on other population groups, initial results do appear encouraging.

Early evidence of the discriminative and predictive validity of the revised scale was provided by studies reporting strong relationships between the scale and measures of depression, and earlier research showed strong relationships between loneliness items and anxiety and self-esteem (Russell 1982).

The revised version of the scale was tested for validity on 162 students, and also using the Beck Depression Inventory. Correlations of 0.32 were obtained with an anxiety index and of 0.62 with the Beck Depression Inventory. The discriminant validity was also assessed by a study of 237 students, with the aim of assessing whether it was measuring a different dimension of well-being to the depression scales. Multivariate analysis was used for this purpose and it was reported that a loneliness index explained an additional 18 per cent of the variance in loneliness scores beyond that accounted for by the mood and personality measures. Concurrent validity was also assessed, and significant associations were reported between solitary activities, having fewer friends and loneliness scores (Russell 1982).

However, the validity of loneliness scales is difficult to assess. In terms of content and face validity, the most face-valid loneliness measures are questions simply asking 'are you lonely?'. This then faces the problem of social desirability bias that could limit validity. Problems with the assessment of criterion validity also exist. Loneliness is not synonymous with isolation. There is an absence of external validity criteria for loneliness. Even ratings by others known to the person are not highly reliable.

The scale reportedly has discriminatory ability and has been used in a number of studies of emotional well-being. Stokes (1985) analysed social-network structure and personality factors in relation to loneliness, using the earlier version of the UCLA, in a sample of 97 male and 82 female students. He reported network density to be the most strongly related to loneliness: people with interconnected networks tend to be less lonely. This may be because they feel more sense of community, of belonging to a group. Extraversion and introversion were also related to loneliness.

Mellor and Edelmann (1988) used the revised UCLA loneliness scale in a study of loneliness in 36 people aged over 65. They found that loneliness was associated with having fewer confidants and with lack of mobility.

Reliability

Studies of the original version (which had a different scoring method of 0 to 3) by Russell *et al.* (1978) and Perlman and Peplau (1981) have reported good reliability for the scale (alpha: 0.94) and evidence of validity, similarly with the revised version (Russell *et al.* 1980; Russell 1982).

The revised scale has a high internal consistency with a coefficient alpha of 0.96, and a second study of 237 students further confirmed the internal consistency of the scale (0.94) and correlations with other relevant items. As for test-retest reliability, Jones (cited in Russell *et al.* 1978) found a correlation of 0.73 over a two-month period in a student sample.

In sum, this scale is the most extensively tested of all the loneliness scales available and results so far are encouraging. The main limitation of testing to date has been its reliance on student subjects who may not be representative of the general population.

7
Measures of life satisfaction and morale

The first population survey of emotional well-being (i.e. life satisfaction and morale) was conducted in 1957 by Gurin *et al.* (1960) in the USA. Respondents were asked: 'Taking all things together, how would you say things are these days – would you say you're very happy, pretty happy or not too happy these days?' Those in the 'not too happy' group were more likely to have psychiatric problems, to be widowed or divorced, to have less education and lower income levels, and to be black. The concept and measurement of well-being, in relation to happiness, life satisfaction and morale, are now receiving increasing attention and more sophisticated measurement scales have been developed, particularly in gerontology. The reason is that indicators of these concepts are useful in assessing the mental health or well-being of people. Life satisfaction, for example, has been related to mental health (Gurin *et al.* 1960; Bradburn 1969).

Measures of well-being are subjective (Campbell 1976). A major methodological problem has been the lack of consistency in the usage of the terms 'happiness', 'life satisfaction' and 'morale' (Stull 1987; Stones and Kozma 1980). While the concepts and measures are related, it has been argued that 'life satisfaction' and 'morale' have a more cognitive component to them, while happiness has a more affective or emotional component (Andrews and McKennel 1980). The cognitive component implies evaluation, while affect refers to the positive/negative feeling. These concepts relating to well-being are not identical, although many researchers continue to treat these concepts as interchangeable (George and Bearon 1980).

Happiness
This has been defined as transitory moods of 'gaiety and elation' that reflect the affect that people feel toward their current state of affairs

(Campbell *et al.* 1976). It has also been defined as the extent to which positive feelings outweigh negative feelings (Bradburn 1969). The latter definition often includes the time dimension of 'the past few weeks'. Happiness implies an affective mood or state.

Life satisfaction

This generally refers to some overall assessment of one's life or a comparison reflecting some perceived discrepancy between one's aspiration and achievement (Campbell *et al.* 1976). Questions regarding overall assessment as well as satisfaction with certain domains are asked. Some explicit or implicit comparison group is usually involved ('compared to others'). In this regard, satisfaction suggests a cognitive process.

Morale

This is the most poorly defined and measured concept of the three. Kutner *et al.* (1956) defined morale as 'a continuum of responses to life and living problems that reflect the presence or absence of satisfaction, optimism, and expanding life perspectives.' Lawton (1972, 1975) has defined morale as a basic sense of satisfaction with oneself, a feeling that there is a place in the environment for oneself, and an acceptance of what cannot be changed. George (1979) and Stones and Kozma (1980) define morale as 'courage, discipline, confidence, enthusiasm'.

Lohmann (1977) has shown that many of the major scales of well-being in use are correlated quite substantially. This suggests that all measures are directed towards tapping a common underlying construct. Many of the questions in the scales are similar, accounting for their overlap and intercorrelations. This is particularly true for the Philadelphia Geriatric Center Morale Scale (see page 159) and Neugarten's Life Satisfaction Index A (see page 152). McKennell (1978) has argued that happiness and life-satisfaction measures differentially tap cognitive and affective components, and that correlations between these measures result from loadings on underlying factors that the measures have in common.

   The main difficulty for researchers in this area is that of conceptualization – whether or not the dimensions of well-being employed reflect attitudes, personality or mood states and whether or not well-being really is represented by some combination of these.

   Two other issues are of concern. Smith (1979) has stated that there appears to be seasonal variation in the global measure of happiness, with happiness highest in the spring, declining in the summer and autumn and dropping to its lowest point in winter. The other is the possibility of positivity bias among some sample members: some people may be reluctant to admit the extent of any unhappiness they may feel on the basis of the assumption that it is socially desirable to be 'happy'.

A further concept which requires inclusion here is self-esteem. Self-esteem is conceptualized slightly differently by psychologists and sociologists. Psychologists refer to self-esteem in relation to a sense of self-worth – a belief that one is a person of value, accepting personal strengths and weaknesses (Wells and Marwell 1976; Rosenberg 1965; Coopersmith 1967). Self-esteem is therefore a self-evaluation. Related concepts include self-regard, self-acceptance, self-concept and self-image. These are all based upon the individual's assessment and evaluation of him/herself (Crandall 1973; Wells and Marwell 1976). High self-esteem is viewed as a component of mental health. Self-concept is the cognitive component of the self and consists of individuals' perceptions of themselves (i.e. what I am really like?). In sociology, the critical role of social interaction and the significance of others in developing self-esteem and its maintenance is emphasized (Wylie 1974). In relation to health and illness, Wilson Barnett (1981) has reviewed the literature on recovery from disease, principally heart surgery, and reports that negative images of the self are associated with delayed or poor recovery.

Available evidence suggests that positive self-esteem is an important component of general assessment of life (Andrews and Withey 1976). Self-esteem may become increasingly salient with the transition from middle to old age (Schwartz 1975). Most self-esteem theorists suggest, with some evidence, that self-esteem is developed and maintained through a successful process of personal interaction and negotiation with the environment (Wells and Marwell 1976; Rosenberg 1965). As successful negotiations are less likely in later life, self-esteem among older people is less likely to be positive. Schwartz (1975) has thus defined self-esteem as the essential component of quality of life for the aged. If age changes are to be expected, the impact of an intervention could become confounded with developmental changes over time. Evidence is limited and there is no reason why a sensitive measure to assess the impact of interventions should not be attempted. As self-esteem is a dimension of life satisfaction, morale and happiness, scales of self-esteem are reviewed at the end of this chapter.

Global items

The first set of measures to be discussed are the commonly used global measures of happiness and life satisfaction. The choice of whether to measure satisfaction or happiness, or both, depends on the interests of the researcher, as they tap different dimensions of affect and cognition.

Life satisfaction, morale and happiness are all global concepts, referring to life as a whole rather than to specific aspects of it. Global measures are of relevance in assessing well-being, although they may be of limited utility in evaluative research (George and Bearon 1980). Carp (1977) cautions against drawing policy relevant inferences from data which do not reveal why and with what people are satisfied. Item specific measures are an alternative (e.g. housing satisfaction in evaluating effect of relocation) (Campbell *et al.* 1976; Andrews and Withey 1976). Global and item-specific measures are appropriate for different research questions.

One of the advantages of overall global questions is brevity: one or two questions rather than a whole battery. However, a positivity bias, for example, respondents' desire to be socially desirable, can be obtained with short items. Also short items lack sensitivity and therefore are of limited predictive value in longitudinal studies. The effect of question order with such items has been relatively unexplored, although the National Opinion Research Centre found that placing a question about marital happiness immediately before a global question of happiness resulted in a more positive response on global happiness (Smith 1979).

A review of the literature indicates that well-being has been measured by four major scales or global items: Life Satisfaction A (Neugarten *et al.* 1961); Bradburn Affect-Balance Scales (Bradburn and Caplovitz 1965; Bradburn 1969); Philadelphia Geriatric Center Morale Scale (Lawton 1975); and global items of happiness and life satisfaction (Robinson and Shaver 1973; Campbell *et al.* 1976; Smith 1979). Other popular scales are the Delighted–Terrible Faces Scale (Andrews and Withey 1976) and the Psychological Well-Being Scale (Dupuy 1978). These will be reviewed in the following sections. For examples of single items, readers are referred to Robinson and Shaver (1973).

The Life Satisfaction Index A (LSIA) and Index B (LSIB)

The Life Satisfaction Indexes A and B were developed by Neugarten *et al.* (1961) in order to produce a relatively short self-report measure of life satisfaction based on respondents' feelings. The aim of these scales is to measure general feelings of well-being in order to identify 'successful' ageing. Several versions of the LSI exist. All are derived from the five dimensions of past and present life from a life-satisfaction rating obtained by a clinical interview: zest and apathy, resolution and fortitude, congruence between desired and achieved goals, positive self-concept and mood tone.

LSIA and LSIB were first developed in 1956 on the basis of four rounds of interviews on the subject of life satisfaction, with people aged 50–70, based on a stratified probability sample of middle- and working-class people residing in Kansas City. A second sample was interviewed aged 70-90 two years later, based on a quota sample (overall total 177).

All versions of the index are easily administered and rest on a substantial amount of empirical support. The problem with the scale is its global nature which poses uncertainty about what is being measured. Scale A has been further criticized by Liang (1984) for failing to measure transitory effects.

Content

Scales A and B differ only slightly in content but greatly in form. Life Satisfaction Index A has a check-list of 20 items, statements with which the respondent either agrees or disagrees. Life Satisfaction Index B has 17 open-ended questions that are given a score based upon the content of the answers. The two instruments can be used together or separately (Neugarten *et al.* 1961). Index A has been used more frequently than B, probably due to ease of administration and quantification of structured items.

The original LSIA consists of 20 items (12 positive and 8 negative). A second version, which is infrequently used, consists of 12 questions using a three-point response scale. A third version, adapted by Wood *et al.* (1969) contains 13 of the original 20 items. Another version uses 18 items. An advantage of Scales A and B, and the shorter versions of A, is that they have positive and negative items.

A wide variety of content areas are tapped by each of these scales, for example, ranging from happiness to satisfaction with level of activity. Some items reflect back over past lives or involve comparing the present with the past, as well as assessment of the present.

Respondents agree or disagree with the items on Scale A; each positive response receives a score of 1. Examples of Scale A items are:

Positive items
I have had more luck in my life than most people
These are the best years of my life
The things I do today are as interesting to me as they ever were

Negative items
This is the dreariest time of my life
Most of the things I do are boring and monotonous
Compared to other people I get down in the dumps too often

Examples of the open-ended items on B are:

Positive
What are the best things about being the age you are now?
(1=positive answer; 0=nothing good about it)

What is the most important thing in your life at the moment?
(2=anything outside of self, or pleasant interpretation of future; 1=hanging on;
keeping health or job; 0=getting out of present difficulty, or nothing now, or
reference to past).

Negative
Do you wish you could see more of your close friends than you do, or would you
like more time to yourself?
(2=OK as it is; 0=wish could see more of friends; 0=wish more time to self)

How much unhappiness would you say you find in your life today?
(2=almost none; 1=some; 0=a great deal).

Scoring

Scores are summed over all the items; thus ratings of each dimension are
combined. The criticism of this is that the separate dimensions are
confounded.

There are two scoring methods for the LSI. In the original method, a
two-point agree/disagree response choice rated dissatisfaction as 0 and
satisfaction as 1. Analysis of 'undecided' responses then led to the use of a
three-point scale, rating satisfaction as 2, uncertain as 1, and dissatisfaction
as 0 (Wood *et al.* 1969).

The mean LSI score varies slightly between studies, reflecting different
population bases. In the original sample the mean score was 12.4, with a
standard deviation of 4.4. Others have reported mean scores ranging
between 11.6 (a sample of elderly residents in rural Kansas) to 14.1 (a
sample of British males in manual and professional occupations) (see
review by George and Bearon 1980). For the 13-item three-point response
version, Harris (1975) reported mean scores of 26.7 for adults aged under 64
and 24.4 for those aged 65+.

Several studies using factor analysis and multiple regression models have
confirmed the multidimensional nature of the scale and have questioned
the original conceptual formulation (Hoyt and Creech 1983). In view of its
multidimensionality the use of a single score blurs the relationships
between the items and it should instead be used as a series of subscales.
Comparisons require caution, given the different scoring systems used.

Validity

Neugarten *et al.* (1961) reported a correlation of 0.55 between LSIA and the
original clinical life satisfaction rating instrument of 0.55. As the former
was derived from the latter, this is not a sound test of the validity of the
scale. The correlation of scores on LSIA with judges' ratings was 0.52, and
the correlation of LSIB with judges' ratings was 0.59. Details of these and

of the item analysis employed to derive the index items have been described by Neugarten *et al.* (1961).

Criterion validity was established by assessments by a clinical psychologist, although these were 18–22 months after the fourth interview on 80 remaining sample members and were of questionable value. The correlation between judges' and clinical ratings was 0.64 which was regarded as satisfactory in view of these problems.

Correlations between the LSIA and the Affect-Balance Scale and the Philadelphia Geriatric Center Morale Scale have been reported as 0.66 and 0.76 respectively (Bild and Havighurst 1976; Lohmann 1977).

Bowling and Browne (1991), in an interview study of 662 people aged 85 and over living at home in London, reported that the correlation between Neugarten's Life Satisfaction Scale A and the Delighted–Terrible Faces Scale was –0.65, and with the General Health Questionnaire (which assesses mainly anxiety and depression) was –0.47 (i.e. greater life satisfaction was associated with low anxiety and depression). A similar study by the authors (unpublished) of almost 300 people aged 65 and over living at home in Essex, and of almost 400 people aged 65 to 85 living at home in London between reported correlations and Neugarten's Scale and the Delighted–Terrible Faces Scale and the General Health Questionnaire of –0.24 and –0.47 (Essex) and –0.57 and –0.41 (London) respectively. Although the correlations with the General Health Questionnaire were very similar for the three studies (–0.41 to –0.47), it is uncertain why the correlations with the Faces scale vary between studies (–0.24 to –0.65), or should be weaker with the younger elderly groups. High correlations between these scales would not be expected as they tap different dimensions of well-being, although overlap would be (as is demonstrated).

Other inconsistencies using the scale have been reported. For example, although the original authors reported that LSIA did not correlate with demographic factors, other studies have indicated that it does. In particular positive correlations with socio-economic status have been reported by a number of authors (see review by McDowell and Newell, 1987).

Reliability

Internal consistency coefficients in various studies range from 0.70 to 0.76 (Dobson *et al.* 1979) to around 0.79 (Wood *et al.* 1969; Stock and Okun 1982), depending upon the version used.

Reliability ratings were made by seven pairs of judges who rated descriptions of 177 cases. The coefficient of correlation between the pairs of ratings was 0.79. For the 177 cases life-satisfaction scores for Scale A ranged from 8 to 25, with a mean of 17.8, and a standard deviation of 4.6. There was no significant difference with sex (Neugarten *et al.* 1961).

This author (Bowling) has found problems with the scale which affect reliability. The final item 'In spite of what people say, the life of the average person is getting worse not better' is often received with puzzlement about a stereotyped 'average person'. This item assumes agreement over an 'average' person. Moreover, respondents' agreement with this item does not inform us whether their own lives are getting 'worse not better'. Also, it makes the scale too diverse in the number of different dimensions of life satisfaction covered. Two other items also require refinement: 'I feel my age but it does not bother me' – this is difficult for respondents to reply to if they feel their age, but it does bother them; and 'Compared to other people my age, I look smart when I am dressed to go out' – this is difficult to reply to in the case of respondents who are housebound or who live in institutions and do not go out. In the author's study of people aged 85 and over in London and aged 65 and over in Essex and London, the alpha reliability coefficients for the scale ranged from alpha 0.73 to 0.80; and the split-half reliability coefficients ranged from 0.65 to 0.74.

The Life Satisfaction Index Z 13-item version (LSIZ)

Validity, reliability and sensitivity

Wood *et al.* (1969) have derived a 13-item version of Scale A, known as LSIZ, which is probably the most popular, and applications are numerous.

Moderate correlations were obtained between the LSIZ and a scale of social engagement (0.49) and between the LSIZ and the Symptoms of Anxiety and Depression Scale (0.49), the latter suggesting that the scales assess some common aspect of well-being (Wood *et al.* 1969). The 13-item LSIZ has been extensively used in the USA. It was used by Usui *et al.* (1985) in a community survey of people aged 60+ in Jefferson County, Kentucky. The authors reported a correlation of –0.22 between number of physical health problems and life satisfaction, and similar correlations with various social activities, income level and life satisfaction; these were confirmed by multiple regression analysis. In contrast to Morgan *et al.* (1987), in a study of over 1500 people aged 65+ in Nottinghamshire in the UK, they reported that older respondents had higher life-satisfaction scores. Morgan *et al.* reported that the average score was 17 for people aged 65–74 and 16.4 for people aged 75+; life satisfaction was significantly lower for those aged 75+.

The LSIZ was used by Kozma and Stones (1987), along with other measures of well-being, in a study of 150 people in acute psychiatric or community psychiatric wards, aged between 50 and 82, in Newfoundland. Correlations between the LSIZ and the Philadelphia Geriatric Center Morale Scale (PGCMS) were reported to be high (0.74). The authors reported that the LSIZ was able to correctly identify 72 per cent of the community-hospital or acute-ward samples, and PGCMS correctly identified 74 per cent. A scale of social desirability was also used, and the authors reported that controlling for social desirability did not enhance the construct validity of the well-being scales.

Wood *et al.* (1969) reported that the refined 13-item version of the Index shows a split-half reliability of 0.79. Edwards and Klemmack (1973) reported an internal consistency reliability coefficient of 0.90.

It has been found to be sensitive to change in a study of participation in community programmes (Wylie 1970). As it was developed for use with older people, it is appropriate for use with that population. The scoring for this version of the scale ranges from 0 to 26; item scores are satisfaction: 2; dissatisfaction: 1; don't know: 1.

Although the scales are satisfactory in terms of standard tests of reliability and validity, their global and multidimensional nature do pose problems. The issue is what is being predicted? However, these scales are the most commonly used to measure well-being in gerontological research (Larson 1978; Stull 1987).

The Affect-Balance Scale (ABS)

Bradburn (1969) described the Affect-Balance Scale as an indicator of happiness or general psychological well-being. It is not concerned with detecting psychiatric or psychological disorders. Bradburn and Caplovitz (1965) hypothesized that subjective well-being could be indicated by a person's position on two independent dimensions: positive and negative affect. Well-being is expressed as the balance between these two. Thus positive factors can compensate for negative feelings. The scale was developed by Bradburn and Caplovitz (1965) on the basis of a sample of 2,006 adults in Illinois, and by Bradburn (1969), in a revision, on 2,787 adults of mixed socio-economic and ethnic groups based on five probability random samples in Detroit, Chicago, Washington and ten large US cities. Respondents were reinterviewed twelve weeks apart for the latter study.

This scale has been subjected to a great deal of analysis (Knapp 1976). Originally 12 items, it is now composed of 10 items, 5 referring to 'positive affect', and 5 referring to 'negative affect'. The two subscales are independent, although both correlate with happiness (Bradburn 1969). Balance refers to the balance between positive and negative effect reflected by an individual's score on the scale (the balance is the result of an additive process). However, this scale is also confounded by items referring to activation (e.g. the item 'excited' or 'interested' in something). Additionally some of the items also appear to measure accomplishments. The scale is self-administered.

Content

The wording of the questions appears to have varied between studies. Bradburn specified that the time referent should be 'the past few weeks' (originally 'the past week'). Others have used 'the past few months' or even no time referent (see review by McDowell and Newell 1987).

An advantage of using the scale is that some items refer to positive psychological states, reflecting the recent interest in positive health. Examples of scale items are:

Positive items include:

On top of the world because someone complimented you.
Things going your way.
Excited, interested in something.
Pleased about having accomplished something.

Negative items include:

Too restless to sit long in chair (anxiety).
Depressed or very unhappy.
Upset because someone criticized you.
Very lonely, remote from people.
Bored.

Scoring

Replies are dichotomous (yes/no). Differential weights were tested but did not significantly alter the results and so are not used.

The overall score on the ABS involves a complex calculation. Sub-scale scores are determined independently by summing scores for the five items in each sub-scale. The two items in each sub-scale with the lowest frequencies are then combined, so sub-scale scores range from 0 to 4; the Negative Affect score is then subtracted from that of Positive Affect, and the resulting overall score transformed to range from +1 to +9 by the addition of a constant (+5). The contribution of each psychological construct to the overall score is determined by the number of items measuring the construct. The ABS total score reflects positive and negative affect nearly equally because ABS items are equally divided between these constructs. Results from studies using this scale, and those using the General Well-Being Schedule, suggest that about 10 per cent of the general population may experience a strong sense of positive well-being.

Validity

Correlations with other measures (testing for validity) are around 0.66;

this was achieved with an 18-item version of Neugarten's LSIA (Bild and Havighurst 1976). A review of the scale by George and Bearon (1980) reports inter-scale correlations with other morale scales and an 18-item version of the LSIA of between 0.61 and 0.64.

Cherlin and Reeder (1975) have criticized the scale, suggesting that the two-dimensional structure is not correct. They suggested that there is a third component (activation level) included (e.g. 'particularly excited or interested in something'). Borgatta and Montgomery (1987) have also argued that some items also seem to be measuring instrumental aspects (e.g. accomplishments).

It has been reported to be sensitive to change (Bradburn 1969). The scale was used by Berkanovic et al. (1988) in an interview study of distress and help-seeking among 950 respondents in Los Angeles. The authors found no relationship between distress and use of medical care, although they reported that the distressed reported more illnesses. Significant differences on scale scores by sex of respondents have been reported (Kushman and Lane 1980). Possibly the most well-known application of the scale was by Berkman (1971) in the Alameda County survey, although she only used eight of the items. She reported a correlation of 0.48 with a 20-item index of neurotic traits.

Reliability

Internal consistency (inter-item) correlations range from 0.47 to 0.73 for the positive scale and from 0.48 to 0.73 for the negative scale (Cherlin and Reeder 1975; Warr 1978). Inter-scale correlations were modest at 0.24 to 0.26 (Warr 1978).

Bradburn (1969) tested the scale for reliability and reported a test-retest correlation of 0.76 three days apart; for nine items associations exceeded 0.90 and for the item 'excited or interested' the test-retest correlation was 0.86.

In sum, it has acceptable levels of validity and reliability and has been found to be applicable for use with older people, although it was not developed specifically as a measure for them. It is easily administered. George and Bearon (1980) rate it as the best measure of affect (frequency of experienced feelings and kinds of reported feelings).

The Philadelphia Geriatric Center Morale Scale

This scale and its revised version were developed on the basis of the assumption that well-being is multidimensional (Lawton 1972; 1975). Lawton viewed morale in terms of general well-being. The scale also takes into account two other properties: applicability to older, institutionalized populations, and optimal scale length allowing reliability without respondent fatigue (Knapp 1976). A preliminary version of the scale with 41 items was tested on 300 people, with an average age of 78. The scale originally contained 22 items, but with subsequent analyses was revised and now contains 17 (Morris and Sherwood 1975; Lawton 1975). It was developed for use with older people and is therefore appropriate for these populations. It is easily administered and can be self- or interviewer-administered.

Content

The reduced items obtain three major dimensions: agitation (6 items), attitude towards own ageing (5 items) and lonely dissatisfaction (6 items). Examples of scale items are:

How often do you feel lonely?
I see enough of my friends and relatives.
I am as happy now as when I was younger.
Life is hard for me much of the time.

Scoring

One point is scored for each response indicating high morale. Most items are dichotomously coded. The scale can be treated as three subscales or as an overall scale. Liang and Bollen (1983) have reviewed the various scoring methods.

The range of scores is from 0 (low) to 17 (high), with higher scores indicating greater morale.

Validity

Correlations testing for validity with Neugarten's scales (reported earlier) vary with Neugarten's various indexes from 0.57 to 0.79 (Lawton 1972; Lohmann 1977).

The scale has been criticized by Borgatta and Montgomery (1987) because it includes measures of happiness and life satisfaction; this is alleged to be questionable in a scale purporting to measure 'morale'. This confusion, they argue, is made even more problematic by the use of different time referents (e.g. 'I am as happy now as when I was younger' and 'How satisfied are you with your life today?'). To be fair to the developers of the scale, they did claim to define the concept of morale in terms of general well-being.

There is limited evidence of sensitivity to change (reports exist by Kalson (1976) and Morris (1975)). It has been reported that the scale is able to discriminate between social groups.

The PGCMS has had numerous applications, one of which, using the 17-item version, was by Ward *et al.* (1984). They excluded two items that they were already measuring in a series of questions about social integration: 'How often do you feel lonely?' and 'I see enough of my friends and relatives'. They used the scale with a sample of people, average age 70.6, living in Albany–Schenectady–Troy, New York, and reported that morale was associated with satisfaction with frequency of contact with others.

It was also used by Noelker and Harel (1978) in their survey of 14 nursing-home residents in the USA. The average age of respondents was 81. The authors reported that twice as many residents who desired to live in the homes had high morale scores (mean: 12.98; standard deviation 4.25), compared to residents who desired to live elsewhere (mean: 10.33; standard deviation 4.96). Morale was also best predicted by functional health status: 39 per cent of the variance in morale scores was explained by self-rated health.

Reliability

Lawton (1972) reported a split-half reliability coefficient of 0.74, a coefficient of internal consistency of 0.81, and test-retest reliability coefficients ranging from 0.75 (after three months) to 0.91 (after five weeks).

Factor analysis has been carried out by Lawton (1975), replicating work carried out by others. Seventeen items formed three factors: agitation (6 items), attitude towards one's own ageing (5 items) and lonely dissatis-faction (6 items). They provided alpha internal consistency coefficients of between 0.81 and 0.85. Lawton recommended that these 17 items be referred to as the 'revised PGC Morale scale'.

In sum, the scale has acceptable levels of reliability and validity and is widely believed to be the superior of the existing life-satisfaction and morale scales. The criticism of it is that the inclusion of items measuring both happiness and satisfaction is questionable, given the earlier definition of morale (Stull 1987).

Delighted–Terrible Faces (D–T) Scale

A less widely applied scale is the Delighted–Terrible Faces Scale (Andrews and Withey 1976). This is an affective evaluation of quality of life which involves a cognitive evaluation and some degree of positive/negative feeling (affect).

The D–T Scale was developed in response to the recognition of deficiencies in other scales. Andrews and Withey (1976) report that a survey of well-being by Campbell *et al.* (1976) reported that a half to two-thirds of respondents selected one of the two most satisfied categories presented to them. They felt that this concentration at the 'satisfied' end of the scale posed statistical and conceptual problems. The inclusion of seven faces on the D–T scale was an attempt to reduce the skew of distributions and improve discrimination between respondents. They also offered a neutral face, as they felt it was important for respondents to 'opt out' if none of the faces represented their feelings. The faces show clear expressions and can be regarded as 'labelled' (each face is represented by an alphabetical letter, ranging from A (delighted) to G (terrible)). This was seen as an improvement on scales which are laid out along a single dimension with only the end categories labelled, leaving the respondent to infer the appropriate meanings for the intermediate categories.

Content

Respondents are shown seven faces ranging from wide smiles to turned-down mouths. They are told: 'Here are some faces expressing various feelings (delighted, pleased, mostly satisfied, mixed, mostly dissatisfied, unhappy, and terrible). Below each is a letter. Which face comes closest to expressing how you feel about..?' (specific items and/or 'life as a whole' are asked about). Examples of items which can be included, and which explain 50–62 per cent of the variance in evaluations of life, are self-accomplishment and problem handling, family life, income, fun and enjoyment, accommodation, family togetherness, time to do things one wants to, non-work activities, national government activities, quality of local goods and services, health status and employment.

Andrews and Withey advise researchers to select study-specific items. They have published a wide selection of items which can be incorporated within a scale.

Scoring

The seven faces are given scores from 1 (delighted) to 7 (terrible). While item responses can be summed, each item can also be analysed independently. The latter is more valid given the lack of information about appropriate weighting of items.

A study of 662 people aged 85+ in the East End of London by Bowling and Browne (1991) reported that the D–T Faces Scale was fairly skewed, with about a quarter of respondents choosing the terrible faces, while over half selected a delighted face. Research on stroke patients in the UK by Anderson (1988) also found the measure to be skewed, with 19 per cent of respondents choosing a terrible face and two-thirds choosing a delighted face. However, both studies reported good acceptance of the scale by respondents.

Reproduced with permission from Andrews and Withey, *Social Indicators of Well-being: Americans' Perceptions of Life Quality*.

Validity and reliability

The authors of the scale compared the D–T scale with other similar scales and presented evidence that it was a more valid measure than most other scales assessed; the exception was a visually complex 'circles' scale: different circles had varying numbers of plus signs (these represented good things in life) and minus signs (which represented bad things in life) displayed within them; respondents choose the circles which represent their feelings. Other scales assessed by the authors included a ladder scale in which respondents rated life satisfaction via the ladder rungs; a visual analogue scale with boxes at intervals along the line which represented statements about life satisfaction (delighted–pleased–mostly satisfied–mixed (about equally satisfied and dissatisfied)–mostly dissatisfied–unhappy–terrible), and Bradburn's Affect-Balance Scale. The results are too complex to present here as Andrews and Withey (1976) presented them in model form but are reported in detail by the authors. Few studies using the scale have been published.

It was previously reported by Bowling and Browne (in press) (see section on Neugarten Life Satisfaction Scales, page 155), that, on the basis of their samples of elderly people living at home in London and Essex, the correlations between the D–T Faces Scale and Neugarten's Life Satisfaction Scale A fluctuated fairly widely from weak to moderate: from –0.24 to –0.65 (the correlations were in the expected direction – the minus sign reflects the direction of the scoring).

Further analyses (unpublished) of these studies by Bowling and Browne showed reliability coefficients of around alpha 0.80; inter-item correlations were weak to moderate, ranging from 0.30 to 0.59 between studies.

Apart from the original work by Andrews and Withey, which reported good reliability and validity, there have been few published studies reporting usage of this scale.

The (Psychological) General Well-Being Schedule (GWBS)

The General Well-Being Schedule, sometimes called the Psychological General Well-Being Index (PGWB), is a concise multidimensional indicator of subjective feelings of well-being and distress. It was designed for use in the US Health and Nutrition Examination Survey (Dupuy 1978).

The GWBS Index was developed with the aim of providing an index that could be used to measure self-reports of intrapersonal affective or emotional states reflecting a sense of subjective well-being or distress.

Populations norm were provided by the national Health and Nutrition Examination Survey (HNS). The most well-known application is the modified version incorporated into the Rand Mental Health Inventory, based on a large community sample of people aged 14–60+ (Brook *et al.* 1979a; 1979b). The Rand Health Insurance Survey provided the most recent national reference standards for the GWBS in the USA: 71 per cent of adults fell into the 'positive well-being' category (scores 73–110), 15.5 per cent showed moderate distress (scores of 61–72), and 13.5 per cent were classified as experiencing 'severe distress' (scores of 0–60). Fifteen of the GWBS items were retained for use in the final version of the Rand Mental Health Inventory. Brook *et al.* (1979a; 1979b) have extensively reviewed the scale.

Content

The initial draft of the instrument contained 68 items, 18 of which were used for the US HNS; these were referred to as the General Well-Being Schedule. The index now contains 22 items. The 22 items include indicators of both positive and negative affect. It is a self-administered questionnaire; administration time is 12 minutes.

It includes items for six states of being. The subscales used to measure these six states contain three to five items each. The six sub-scales are anxiety (e.g. bothered by nervousness; generally tense; anxious, worried, upset; relaxed, at ease versus highly strung; felt under strain, stress or pressure); depressed mood (e.g. felt depressed; felt downhearted and blue; sad, discouraged, hopeless); positive well-being (e.g. general spirits; happy, satisfied with personal life; interesting daily life; felt cheerful, lighthearted); self-control (e.g. in firm control; afraid of losing control; felt emotionally stable, sure of self); general health (e.g. bothered by illness, bodily disorders, or aches and pains; healthy enough to do things; concerned, worried about health); and vitality (e.g. energy, pep; waking feeling fresh, rested; felt active, vigorous versus dull, sluggish; felt tired, worn-out, used up).

The frame of reference for questions is 'during the last month'. The first 14 questions have six different response choices; and four questions use rating scales, defined by adjectives at each end. Examples of questions are:

How have you been feeling in general *(during the past month)?*

In excellent spirits

In very good spirits
I have been up and down in spirits a lot
In low spirits mostly
In very low spirits

How happy, satisfied, or pleased have you been with your personal life *(during the past month)?*

Extremely happy – could not have been more satisfied or pleased
Very happy
Fairly happy
Satisfied ... pleased
Somewhat dissatisfied
Very dissatisfied.

How concerned or worried about your health have you been *(during the past month)?*

| 0 | 1 | 2 | 3 | 4 | 5 | 6 | 7 | 8 | 9 | 10 |

Not concerned
at all

Very
concerned

Scoring

The first 14 questions have six response choices which are scored on a scale of 0 to 5. A value of 0 is allocated for the most negative response and 5 for the most positive response (rating scales are also used; see above). The range of scores is from 0 to 110, and the range for the sub-scales is from 0 to 15, or 20 to 25. The overall score or sub-scale scores can be used for analysis. Dupuy proposed that scores of 0–60 reflect 'severe distress', 61–72 'moderate distress', while 73 to 110 represent 'positive well-being'.

Validity

Fazio's (1977) study of 195 students found that the GWBS correlated moderately with interviewers' ratings of depression (0.47); and that the average correlation of the GWBS and six other depression scales was 0.69, and 0.64 with three anxiety scales. Fazio (1977) and Ware *et al.* (1979) also reported criterion correlations between the GWBS and interviewers' ratings generally ranging between 0.65 and 0.90.

Edwards *et al.* (1978) showed that psychiatric patients achieved different scores in comparison with national population norms provided by the HNS. The scale was also sensitive enough to detect the progress over three weeks of the 21 psychiatric day patients in their study. Kammann and Flett

(1983) reported a correlation of 0.74 between the GWBS scale and their 96-item scale of general happiness and well-being (the Affectometer).

On the basis of the US HNS data, Dupuy (1978) and Wan and Livieratos (1977) reported factor analyses of the GWBS which showed three factors which explained 51 per cent of the variance: anxiety, tension and depression; health and energy; and positive well-being or life satisfaction.

Reliability

Extensive scaling and tests of reliability and validity were carried out on 1,209 respondents. A six-factor solution was produced. Internal consistency coefficients for the six sub-scales ranged between 0.72 and 0.88. Test-retest reliability produced good results (with the exception of a lowered test-retest coefficient of 0.50 when the interval was extended from one week to one month). Test-retest reliability coefficients ranged from 0.50 to 0.86, with a median of 0.66.

These results were based on a wide range of studies from samples of students to the large sample of adults participating in the Rand Health Insurance Study. They have been reviewed by Dupuy (1984). Test-retest reliability coefficients of 0.68 and 0.85 for two sub-samples within the US HNS were reported by Monk (1981). It is difficult to know whether the lower correlations reflect the instability of the instrument or changes in individuals. The same data reported internal consistency coefficients of 0.93 on the basis of analyses of 6,913 people. Fazio (1977) reported internal consistency coefficients of 0.91 for males and 0.95 for females; and correlations among sub-scores ranging from 0.16 to 0.72. Ware *et al.*'s (1979) review reported three studies using the GWBS which found internal consistency coefficients of over 0.90. However, Edwards *et al.* (1978) reported a coefficient of 0.69.

This is a scale with good test results on the whole. One advantage of this scale is that it avoids reference to physical symptoms of emotional distress and so avoids problems of interpretation. Fluctuations in test-retest reliability may be problematic in assessing individuals. A major disadvantage is that most of the validation studies of it are unpublished, although these have been thoroughly reviewed by Brook *et al.* (1979a; 1979b).

SCALES OF SELF-ESTEEM

Among the most popular and commonly used measures of self-esteem are: the Self-Esteem Scale (Rosenberg 1965); the Tennessee Self-Concept Scale (Fitts 1965); and the Self-Esteem Inventory (Coopersmith 1967). Several other popular scales have been reviewed by Crandall (1973), Robinson and Shaver (1973), George and Bearon (1980) and by Wylie (1974); the reader is referred to these authors for a more detailed review. Most scales appear to warrant further testing for validity, reliability and sensitivity, and they appear to suffer from concentration on studies of students with little information being provided on their applicability to other population groups.

The Self-Esteem Scale

Rosenberg (1965) described self-esteem as self-acceptance or a basic feeling of self-worth. Rosenberg (1965) developed the Self-Esteem Scale, based on Guttman scaling, for a study of 5,024 students in public schools in New York. Little information exists about the development of the scale. Self-esteem scores were correlated with characteristics such as participation and leadership in school activities. The measure was intended to be brief, global and unidimensional. It has been widely used in varying settings. Evidence suggests it is suitable for use with older people. A study of around 5,000 retired teachers and telephone-company employees by Atchley (1976) reported that men had higher self-esteem than women. Kaplan and Porkorny (1969) in a study of 500 adults in Harris County, Texas, reported that age is unrelated to self-esteem. Ward (1977), on the basis of a study of 323 residents of Madison, Wisconsin, reported that predictors for women's self-esteem were current activities, age-related deprivations and health. Among the elderly (aged 60–92), attitudes towards old age are predictive of self-esteem, and for men income and education are predictive (Ward 1977).

Content

The scale consists of ten items with responses reported along a four-point continuum from 'strongly agree' to 'strongly disagree'. Examples of items are:

I feel that I'm a person of worth, at least on an equal plane with others.
I feel that I have a number of good qualities.
All in all, I am inclined to feel that I am a failure.
I feel I do not have much to be proud of.
At times I think I am no good at all.
On the whole, I am satisfied with myself.
I take a positive attitude toward myself.

Strongly agree (1)/agree (2)/disagree (3)/strongly disagree (4)

Scoring

The measure was designed as a ten-item Guttman scale. The category responses were originally designed to be scored from 0 to 6 (strongly agree to strongly disagree). However, there is no agreement over the method of scoring, and some users score responses dichotomously as 'agree' or 'disagree', and other researchers use a simple summing scale.

Validity

Silber and Tippett (1965) assessed the convergent validity of the scale, and reported item correlations of 0.56 and 0.83. Rosenberg (1965) explicitly chose items for the scale which he felt had face validity. He reported that the scale had acceptable predictive validity in relation to depression levels among volunteers assessed by nurses. Robinson and Shaver (1973) reported that the scale correlated 0.59–0.60 with Coopersmith's Self-Esteem Inventory, depending on the scoring method.

Although there is some evidence to support the construct validity of the scale (Rosenberg 1965), there is little evidence of its sensitivity to change. Rosenberg (1965), in assessing its construct validity, reported that positive self-esteem was predictive of several social and psychological characteristics, such as reduced shyness, depression and more assertiveness and social activities.

Kaplan and Porkorny (1969) reported two uncorrelated factors which accounted for 45 per cent of the total variance. The items forming the first factor they called 'self-derogation', and they stated that the second factor reflected 'defense of individual worth'. Kohn (1969) reported similar results.

Reliability

Reliability (internal consistency and test-retest) has been shown to be good by Rosenberg (1965) who reported a reproducibility coefficient of 0.92 and a scalability coefficient of 0.72; Ward (1977) reported a coefficient of alpha of 0.74 for internal consistency; Silber and Tippett (1965) reported a test-retest reliability coefficient of 0.85 from administrations of the scale to 28 students with a two-week interval.

In sum, the scale is attractive due to its brevity and simplicity but still requires further testing for validity, reliability and sensitivity to change. Also its method of scoring remains unresolved. It is highly recommended by George and Bearon (1980).

Little recent work has been carried out with the scale and Wylie (1974), in her extensive review of the scale, concludes that it is worthy of further research and development.

The Tennessee Self-Concept Scale

The Tennessee Self-Concept Scale is probably the most popular and most often used scale. It was developed for use in mental health rehabilitation in 1956 and revised in 1965 (Fitts 1965). Fitts (1965; 1972) based the scale on Maslow's theory that individuals who are more self-actualizing are more able to realize their true potentialities and to function in a more creative and effective manner. Fitts saw self-concept related to performance. The person who has a clear, consistent, positive and realistic self-concept will behave in a healthy, confident, constructive and effective way. This is dependent on other things being equal, and this, of course, is not always the case.

The scale was developed from other scales and open-ended items, and from self-descriptions from samples of psychiatric patients and non-patients. These were placed on an internal–external scale. Ninety remaining statements were independently classified by seven clinical psychologists into 15 categories. There was perfect agreement on their negative and positive content. The scale was initially tested on 626 people, aged 12–68.

Administration takes approximately 20 minutes, and is based on self-completion.

Content

The scale consists of 100 self-descriptive items and is fairly complicated. Ninety items are categorized under the following labels: physical self, moral-ethical self, personal self, family self and social self. These labels are divided into statements about internal self-concept: self-identity, self-acceptance and behaviour. The scale is intended to summarize an individual's feeling of self-worth, and the degree to which the image is realistic or deviant. Ninety items tap both an internal and external dimension of self-concept. The remaining ten items form a lie scale and measure defensive responses.

Depending on the intended use, two versions of the scale are available – one for counselling and one for clinical or research purposes.

Details of the scale, reviews of unpublished and published studies and population norms, are available in a purchasable report by Fitts (1965) and in a related series of monographs, which are obtainable from Counselor Recordings and Tests, Box 6184-Acklen Station, Nashville, Tennessee 37212. Its commercial nature prohibits reproduction of more than a few items:

I have a healthy body.
I am satisfied with my moral behaviour.

I am a member of a happy family.
I am as sociable as I want to be.

Completely false (1)/mostly false (2)/partly false and partly true (3)/mostly true (4)/completely true (5)

Scoring

Scoring is complex. A set of scoring templates and a scoring matrix is required. A computerized scoring service is available from the publisher.

The response categories to 90 of the items lie along a five-point continuum, ranging from 'completely false' to 'completely true'. The total score is a positive self-esteem score. The ten remaining items are the self-criticism (lie) scale, consisting of mildly negative statements.

The positive self-esteem score has a potential range of 90–450. Fitts (1965) reported a mean score, on the basis of his original sample of 628 adults, of 345.57.

Validity

Correlations demonstrating convergent validity, discriminant and predictive validity have been reported by Fitts (1965) and Thompson (1972). Correlations with an anxiety scale of –0.70 suggest the convergent validity of the scale (Fitts 1965), this has been confirmed by Thompson (1972). Fitts (1965) also reports a correlation of 0.68 with a scale of positive affect.

Vincent (1968) undertook a factor analysis of the scale. Self-acceptance and personal self loaded with several similar measures.

Discriminant validity is partly suggested by a correlation of –0.21 with the F scale measure of authoritarianism; and predictive validity is suggested by its ability to distinguish between mental health and psychopathology (Fitts 1965). The scale has been widely used on samples of juveniles and psychiatric patients, as well as normal adults. Self-esteem has been found to be higher among older people than among adults generally (Grant 1966). While there are many variables that correlate significantly with the scale, there are also many that do not (Reed et al. 1980).

Wylie (1974) questions the discriminant validity on the scale on the grounds of lack of sufficient information reported by Fitts (1965) to suggest the validity of the scale. Moreover, Vacchiano and Strauss (1968) reported that their factor analysis of the scale revealed 20 factors.

Applications of the scale do not show a consistent pattern of results to be able to support the definition of self-concept as defined by Fitts (Walsh 1984). There is also little evidence of the scale's sensitivity to change.

Reliability

Test-retest reliability tests show high correlations of 0.92 for the positive self-esteem score and 0.75 for the self-criticism scale over a two-week period in a study of 60 students (Fitts 1965). Wylie (1974) again criticizes Fitts (1965) for lack of sufficient information to make independent judgements about the reliability of the scale. The question of the scale's reliability remains open.

In sum, it appears usable with older people, although the low self-criticism scores obtained by the elderly should make the user cautious (George and Bearon 1980). It is a popular scale but lengthy to administer. The main disadvantage of this scale is its relative inaccessibility: it is a commercial instrument which has to be purchased, and most of the information about its reliability and validity is only available commercially and is limited in detail. Wylie (1974) argues against the use of this scale, despite its popularity.

Self-Esteem Inventory

Coopersmith (1967) defined self-esteem as self-judgements of personal worth, a definition compatible with earlier definitions. The Self-Esteem Inventory measures attitudes towards the self, encompassing several domains: social, academic, family and personal experiences. The scale was devised by five psychologists for use with children who classified items according to high or low esteem to derive a 50-item scale. Items were reduced to 25, after an item analysis based on the responses of 121 children. The correlation of the longer with the shorter version was 0.95. The scale is self-administered and takes approximately ten minutes.

The 50-item scale has an additional 8 lie-scale items (Coopersmith 1967). A similar 25-item version also exists, and this can be used with adults (aged 16+). The version for adults has been published by Robinson and Shaver (1973).

Content

The items consist of short statements which the subject rates as either 'like me' or 'unlike me'. It is multidimensional, covering leadership-popularity, self-derogation, family-parents, and assertiveness-anxiety. Examples are:

I can make up my mind without too much trouble.
I'm a lot of fun to be with.
I'm popular with people my own age.
It's pretty tough to be me.

Things are all mixed up in my life.
I often feel upset about the work I do.
I'm not as nice looking as most people.
If I have something to say, I usually say it.
Things don't usually bother me.

Scoring

The scoring format remains untested. The item responses 'like me' or 'unlike me' are allocated a value and simply summed. A score is derived by multiplying X, the raw score, by 2 on the short scale and 4 on the long scale. A totally positive score is 100 and a totally negative score is 0.

Validity

Convergent-validity correlations between the scale and other self-esteem scales, based again on students, vary widely between 0.02 and 0.60 (Taylor and Reitz 1968; Ziller *et al.* 1969; Crandall 1973). More consistent correlations with the Rosenberg Self-Esteem Scale were reported by Robinson and Shaver (1973), again using students (total: 300): from 0.59 to 0.60. Hoffmeister (1976) compared two sub-scales of the Self-Esteem Questionnaire which he developed with Coopersmith's Self-Esteem Inventory and reported correlations of 0.40 and 0.61.

Discriminant validity correlations range between 0.44 and 0.75 when tested against a social desirability scale (Taylor and Reitz 1968), indicating that there is possible confounding with social desirability.

Correlations have been reported with scales measuring other concepts, which would be expected on theoretical grounds: Campbell (1967) reported a correlation of 0.31 with an achievement test; Boshier (1968) reported a correlation of 0.80 with the scale and liking one's first name; Wiest (1965) reported a correlation of 0.22 between the scale and the reporting of mutual liking between others and self. Not all correlations are in the direction expected. For example, Trowbridge (1970) reported a higher mean on the scale for children who were socioeconomically disadvantaged.

Robinson and Shaver (1973), on the basis of two samples of students (total: 500), carried out two factor analyses of the scale which indicated its multidimensional nature. Four factors emerged: self-derogation, leadership-popularity, family-parents and assertiveness-anxiety. The family-parents factor was reported to be the most stable and least ambiguous.

Kokenes (1974) estimated the validity of the sub-scales by factor analysis of the responses of 7,600 schoolchildren and reported that the four bipolar dimensions obtained were highly congruent with the test's sub-scales.

It is a stable measure over time and thus is not suitable for longitudinal use where changes require measurement (Coopersmith 1967).

Wylie (1974) questions Coopersmith's claims of validity for the scale, on the grounds of the large number of significance tests undertaken in its development and the non-reporting of the actual number of such tests. The number reaching statistical significance at the 0.5 level was unreported, thus making it impossible to estimate the number that could have occurred by chance alone.

Reliability

The scale was originally administered to 87 schoolchildren. Early testing for test-retest reliability reported high coefficients at 0.88 over five weeks and 0.70 over three years, based on the samples of pre-adolescent schoolchildren (Coopersmith 1967). Split-half reliability tests also show high correlations: 0.90 (Taylor and Reitz 1968). Spatz and Johnson (1973) administered the 50-item child version to 600 students and reported internal-consistency coefficients in excess of 0.80. However, internal consistency was reported to be low in another study of 453 college students (Crandall 1973), a probable consequence of its multidimensionality. In sum, the scale appears to have been well researched and is widely used. A major methodological limitation has been its restricted use with samples of students for the testing of the reliability and validity of the adult version.

References

Abelin, T., Brzezinski, Z.J. and Carstairs, V.D.L. (ed.) (1986). *Measurement in Health Promotion and Protection*. Copenhagen, World Health Organization, Regional Office for Europe, European Series no. 22.

Abramson, J.H., Terespolsky, L., Brook, J.G. *et al.* (1965). 'Cornell Medical Index as a health measure in epidemiological surveys.' *British Journal of Preventive and Social Medicine*, 19: 103–10.

Adams, B.N. (1967). 'Interaction theory and the social network.' *Sociometry*, 30: 64–78.

American Psychological Association (1974). *Standards for Educational and Psychological Tests*. Washington, DC: APA.

Anderson, R. (1988). 'The quality of life of stroke patients and their carers' in Anderson, R. and Bury, M. (eds). *Living with Chronic Illness: The Experience of Patients and Their Families*. London, Unwin Hyman.

Anderson, R., Davies, J.K., McQueen, D.V. *et al.* (1989). *Health Behaviour Research and Health Promotion*. Oxford, Oxford University Press.

Anderson, J. Sullivan, F. and Usherwood, T.P. (1990). The Medical Outcomes Study Instruments (MOSI) – use of a new health status measure in Britain. *Family Practice*, 7: 205–218.

Andrews, F.M. and McKennel, A.C. (1980). 'Measures of self-reported well-being: their affective, cognitive and other components.' *Social Indicators Research*, 18: 127–55.

Andrews, F.M. and Withey, S.B. (1976). *Social Indicators of Well-being: Americans' Perceptions of Life Quality*. New York, Plenum Press.

Arfwidsson, L., Elia, G., D'Laurell, B. *et al.* (1974). 'Can self-rating replace doctors' rating in evaluating anti-depressive treatment?' *Acta Psychiatrica Scandinavica*, 50: 16–22.

Atchley, R.C. (1976). 'Selected social and psychological differences between men and women in later life.' *Journal of Gerontology*, 31: 204–11.

Banks, M.H. (1983). 'Validation of the General Health Questionnaire in a young community sample.' *Psychological Medicine*, 13: 349–53.

Bardelli, D. and Saracci, R. (1978). 'Measuring the quality of life in cancer clinical trials: a sample survey of published trials' in Armitage, P. and Bardelli, D. (eds). *Methods and Impact of Controlled Therapeutic Trials in Cancer.* Geneva: Union Internationale Contre le Cancer. Technical Report Series no. 36, 1978: 75–94.

Barrera, M. (1980). 'A method for the assessment of social support networks in community survey research.' *Connections*, 3: 8–13.

——(1981). 'Social support in the adjustment of pregnant adolescent assessment issues' in Gottlieb, B.H. (ed.). *Social Networks and Social Support.* Beverly Hills, Sage Publications.

Barrera, M. and Ainlay, S. (1983). 'The structure of social support: a conceptual and empirical analysis.' *Journal of Community Psychology*, 11: 133–43.

Barrera, M., Baca, L., Christiansen, J. *et al.* (1985). 'Informant corroboration of social support network data.' *Connections*, 8: 9–13.

Beck, A.T. (1970). *Depression: Causes and Treatment.* Philadelphia, University of Pennsylvania Press.

Beck, A.T., Mendelson, M., Mock, J. *et al.* (1961). 'Inventory for measuring depression.' *Archives of General Psychiatry*, 4: 561–71.

Beck, A.T., Steer, R.A. and Garbin, M.G. (1988). 'Psychometric properties of The Beck Depression Inventory: twenty-five years of evaluation.' *Clinical Psychology Review*, 8: 77–100.

Becker, M. (1974). 'The health belief model and personal health behaviour.' *Health Education Monographs*, 2: 326–73.

Bedford, A., Foulds, G.A. and Sheffield, B.F. (1976). 'A new personal disturbance scale (DSSI/SAD).' *British Journal of Social and Clinical Psychology*, 15: 387–94.

Benjamin, S., Decalmer, P. and Haran, D. (1982). 'Community screening for mental illness: a validity study of the General Health Questionnaire.' *British Journal of Psychiatry*, 140: 174–80.

Berg, R.L., Hallauer, D.S. and Berk, S.N. (1976). 'Neglected aspects of the quality of life.' *Health Services Research*, 11: 391–5.

Bergner, M., Bobbitt, R.A., Carter, W.B. *et al.* (1981). 'The Sickness Impact Profile: development and final revision of a health status measure.' *Medical Care*, 19: 787–805.

Bergner, M., Bobbitt, R.A., Kressel, S. *et al.* (1976a). 'The Sickness Impact Profile: conceptual formulation and methodology for the development of a health status measure.' *International Journal of Health Services*, 6: 393–415.

Bergner, M., Bobbitt, R.A., Pollard, W.E. *et al.* (1976b). 'The Sickness Impact Profile: validation of a health status measure.' *Medical Care*, 14: 57–67.

Berkanovic, E., Hurwicz, M.L. and Landsverk, J. (1988). 'Psychological distress and the decision to seek medical care.' *Social Science and Medicine*, 27: 1215–21.

Berkman, L.F. and Syme, S.L. (1979). 'Social networks, host resistance and mortality: a nine-year follow-up study of Alameda County residents.' *American Journal of Epidemiology*, 109: 186–204.

Berkman, P.L. (1971). 'Life stress and psychological well-being: a replication of Langner's analysis in the Midtown Manhattan study.' *Journal of Health and Social Behaviour*, 12: 35–45.

Berwick, D.M., Budman, S., Damico-White, J. *et al.* (1987). 'Assessment of psychological morbidity in primary care: explorations with the General Health Questionnaire.' *Journal of Chronic Diseases*, 40: 71S–79S.

Bild, B.K. and Havighurst, R.J. (1976). 'Life satisfaction.' *Gerontologist*, 16: 70–5.

Billings, A.G. and Moos, R.H. (1981). 'The role of coping responses and social resources in attenuating the impact of stressful life events.' *Journal of Behavioural Medicine*, 4: 139–57.

—— (1982). 'Social support and functioning among community and clinical groups: a panel model.' *Journal of Behavioural Medicine*, 5: 295–311.

Black, S.E., Blessed, J.A., Edwardson, J.A. *et al.* (1990). 'Prevalence rates of dementia in an ageing population: are low rates due to the use of insensitive instruments?' *Age and Ageing*, 19: 84–90.

Blazer, D.G. (1982). 'Social support and mortality in an elderly community population.' *American Journal of Epidemiology*, 115: 684–94.

Blessed, G., Tomlinson, B.E. and Roth, M. (1968). 'The association between quantitative measures of dementia and of senile change in the cerebral grey matter of elderly subjects.' *British Journal of Psychiatry*, 114: 797.

Bombardier, C., Ware, J., Russell, J. *et al.* (1986). 'Auranofin therapy and quality of life in patients with rheumatoid arthritis.' *American Journal of Medicine*, 81: 565–78.

Bond, J. and Carstairs, V. (1982). *Services for the Elderly*. Scottish Health Service Studies no. 42. Edinburgh, Scottish Home and Health Department.

Bond, J., Gregson, B., Atkinson, A. *et al.* (1989). *Evaluation of Continuing Care Accommodation for Elderly People*, vol. 2. *The Randomised Controlled Trial of the Experimental NHS Nursing Homes and Conventional Continuing Care Wards in NHS Hospitals*. Report no. 38, Newcastle upon Tyne, University of Newcastle upon Tyne Health Care Research Unit.

Borgatta, E.F. and Montgomery, R.J.V. (1987). *Critical Issues in Ageing Policy: Linking Research and Values*. Beverly Hills, Sage Publications.

Boshier, R. (1968). 'Self esteem and first names in children.' *Psychological Reports*, 22: 762.

Bowling, A. (1990). 'The prevalance of psychiatric morbidity among people aged 85 and over living at home.' *Social Psychiatry and Psychiatric Epidemiology*, 25: 132–40.

Bowling, A. and Browne, P. (1991). 'Social support and emotional well-being among the oldest old living in London.' *Journal of Gerontology*, 46: S20–32.

Bowling, A. and Cartwright, A. (1982). *Life after a Death: A Study of the Elderly Widowed*. London, Tavistock Press.

Bowling, A. and Charlton, J. (1987). 'Risk factors for mortality after bereavement: a logistic regression analysis.' *Journal of the Royal College of General Practitioners*, 37: 551–4.

Bowling, A. and Formby, J. (1990). *Evaluation of District Health Authority Funded Nursing Homes and Geriatric Wards in City and Hackney*. London, Department of Public Health City and Hackney District Health Authority.

Bowling, A. and Salvage, A. (1986). 'Prevention of residential care among the elderly.' *Community Care*, 13 March: 24–7.

Bowling, A., Edelmann, R., Leaver, J. *et al.* (1989). 'Loneliness, mobility, well-being and social support in a sample of over-65-year-olds.' *Journal of Personality and Individual Differences*, 10: 1189–97.

Bowling, A., Leaver, J. and Hoeckel, T. (1988). *The Needs and Circumstances of People Aged 85+ Living at Home in City and Hackney.* London, Department of Public Health, City and Hackney Health Authority.

Bradburn, N.M. (1969). *The Structure of Psychological Well-being.* Chicago, Aldine Publishing.

Bradburn, N.M. and Caplovitz, D. (1965). *Reports on Happiness: A Pilot Study of Behaviour Related to Mental Health.* Chicago, Aldine Publishing.

Bradwell, A.R., Carmal, M.H. and Whitehead, T.P. (1974). 'Explaining the unexpected: abnormal results of biochemical profile investigations.' *Lancet*, ii: 1071–4.

Brodman, K., Erdman, A.J., Jr, Lorge, I. *et al.* (1953). 'The Cornell Medical Index–Health Questionnaire VI: the relation of patients' complaints to age, sex, race and education.' *Journal of Gerontology*, 8: 339–42.

——(1954). 'The Cornell Medical Index – Health Questionnaire VII: the prediction of psychosomatic and psychiatric disabilities in army training.' *American Journal of Psychiatry*, 111: 37–40.

Brodman, K., Erdmann, A.J., Jr and Wolff, H.G. (1949). *Cornell Medical Index Health Questionnaire.* New York, Cornell University Medical College.

Brodman, K., Van Woerkom, A.J., Jr and Goldstein, L.S. (1959). 'Interpretation of symptoms with a data-processing machine.' *Archives of Internal Medicine*, 103: 776–82.

Brook, R.H., Ware, J.E., Davies-Avery, A. *et al.* (1979a). 'Overview of adult health status measures fielded in Rand's health insurance study.' *Medical Care*, 17 (supplement), 1–131.

—— (1979b). *Conceptualization and Measurement of Health for Adults in the Health Insurance Study*, vol. VIII, Overview. Santa Monica, California, Rand Corporation, R-1987/8-HEW.

Brorsson, B. and Asberg, K.H. (1984). 'Katz Index of Independence in ADL: reliability and validity in short-term care.' *Scandinavian Journal of Rehabilitative Medicine*, 16: 125–32.

Brown, B., Bhrolchain, M. and Harris, T. (1975). 'Social class and psychiatric disturbance among women in an urban population.' *Sociology*, 9: 225–54.

Brown, G.L. and Zung, W.W.K. (1972). 'Depression scales: self or physician rating? A validation of certain clinically observable phenomena.' *Comprehensive Psychiatry*, 13. 361–7.

Brown, J.H., Lewis, M.D., Kazis, E. *et al.* (1984). 'The dimensions of health outcomes: a cross validated examination of health status measurement.' *American Journal of Public Health*, 74: 159–61.

Bucquet, D., Condom, S. and Ritchie, K. (1990). 'The French version of the Nottingham Health Profile: a comparison of item weights with those of the source version.' *Social Science and Medicine*, 30: 829–35.

Burnam, M.A., Wells, K.B., Leake, B. *et al.* (1988). Development of a brief screening instrument for detecting depressive disorders. *Medical Care* 26: 775–789.

Bush, J.W. (1984). 'General health policy model: Quality of well-being (QWB) scale' in Wenger, N.K., Mattson, M.E., Furberg, C.D. *et al.* (eds). *Assessment of Quality of Life in Clinical Trials of Cardiovascular Therapies.* New York, Le Jacq Publ. Co. Inc.

Buxton, M. (1983). 'The economics of heart transplant programmes: measuring the benefits' in Teeling Smith, G. (ed.). *Measuring the Social Benefits of Medicine.* London, Office of Health Economics, 1983.

Byrne, D.G. (1978). 'Cluster analysis applied to self reported depressive symptomatology.' *Acta Psychiatrica Scandinavica,* 57: 1–10.

Caldwell, J.R. (1985). 'Family Environment Scale' in Keyser, D.J. and Sweetland, R.C. (eds). *Test Critiques,* volume II. Kansas City, Missouri, Test Corporation of America.

Caldwell, R.A. and Reinhart, M. (unpublished). *An Empirical Investigation of the Structure of Social Support: An Effort at Concept Clarification.* East Lansing, Michigan State University, Department of Psychology.

Cairl, R.E., Pfeiffer, E., Keller, D.M. *et al.* (1983). 'An evaluation of the reliability and validity of the functional assessment inventory.' *Journal of the American Geriatric Society,* 31: 607–12.

Campbell, A. (1976). 'Subjective measures of wellbeing.' *American Psychologist,* 31: 117–24.

Campbell, A., Converse, P.E. and Rogers, W.L. (1976). *The Quality of American Life.* New York, Russell Sage Foundation.

Campbell, P.B. (1967). 'School and self concept.' *Educational Leadership,* 24: 510–15.

Caplan, G. (1974). *Support Systems and Community Mental Health.* New York, Behavioral Publications.

Carp, F.M. (1977). 'What questions are we asking of whom?' in Nydegger, C.N. (ed.). *Measuring Morale: A Guide to Effective Assessment.* Washington D.C., Gerontology Society.

Carroll, B.J., Fielding, J.M. and Blash, T.G. (1973). 'Depression rating scales: a critical review.' *Archives of General Psychiatry,* 28: 361–6.

Carter, W., Bobbitt, R.A., Bergner, M. *et al.* (1976). 'Validation of an interval scaling: the Sickness Impact Profile.' *Health Services Research,* 11: 516–28.

Cartwright, A. and Anderson, R. (1981). *General Practice Revisited: A Second Study of Patients and Their Doctors.* London, Tavistock Press.

Cassel, J. (1976). 'The contribution of the social environment to host resistance.' *American Journal of Epidemiology,* 104: 107–23.

Cavanaugh, S. (1983). 'The prevalence of emotional and cognitive dysfunction in a general medical population: using the MMSE, GHQ and BDI.' *General Hospital Psychiatry,* 5: 15–24.

Chambers, L.W. (1982). 'The McMaster Health Index Questionnaire (MHIQ): methodologic documentation and report of second generation of investigators.' Hamilton, Ontario, McMaster University, Department of Clinical Epidemiology and Biostatistics.

—— (1984). 'The McMaster Health Index Questionnaire' in Wenger, N.K., Mattson, M.E., Furberg, C.D. *et al.* (eds). *Assessment of Quality of Life in Clinical Trials of Cardiovascular Therapies.* New York, Le Jacq Publ. Co. Inc., 1984.

Chambers, L.W., Haight, M., Norman, G. *et al.* (1987). 'Sensitivity to change and the effect of mode of administration on health status measurement.' *Medical Care,* 25: 470–9.

Chambers, L.W., MacDonald, L.A., Tugwell, P. *et al.* (1982). 'The McMaster Health Index Questionnaire as a measure of quality of life for patients with rheumatoid disease.' *Journal of Rheumatology,* 9: 780–4.

Chambers, L.W., Sackett, D.L., Goldsmith, C.H. *et al.* (1976). 'Development and application of an index of social function.' *Health Services Research*, 11: 430–41.

Charlton, J.R.H., Patrick, D.L. and Peach, H. (1983). 'Use of multivariate measures of disability in health surveys.' *Journal of Epidemiology and Community Health*, 37: 296–304.

Cherlin, A. and Reeder, L.G. (1975). 'The dimensions of psychological well being: a critical review.' *Sociological Methods Research*, 4: 189–214.

Chiange, C.L. (1965). *An Index of Health: Mathematical Models*. Washington: US Government Printing Office, PHS Publication no. 1000, Series 2, no. 5.

Cleary, P.D., Goldberg, D.M., Kessler, L.G. *et al.* (1982). 'Screening for mental disorder among primary care physicians: usefulness of the General Health Questionnaire.' *Archives of General Psychiatry*, 39: 837–40.

Coates, A., Gebski, V., Stat, M. *et al.* (1987). 'Improving the quality of life during chemotherapy for advanced breast cancer.' *New England Journal of Medicine*, 317: 1490–5.

Cobb, S. (1976). 'Social support as a moderator of life stress.' *Psychosomatic Medicine*, 38: 300–14.

Cochrane, A.L. and Holland, W.W. (1971). 'Validation of screening procedures.' *British Medical Bulletin*, 27: 3–8.

Cohen, C.I., Teresi, J. and Holmes, D. (1987). 'Social networks and mortality in an inner-city elderly population.' *International Journal of Ageing and Human Development*, 24: 257–69.

Cohen, S., Mermelstein, R., Karmack, T. *et al.* (1985). 'Measuring the functional components of social support' in Saronson, I.S. and Saronson, B.R. (eds). *Social Support: Theory, Research and Applications*. Boston, Martinus Nijhoff.

Collin, C., Wade, D.T., Davies, D. *et al.* (1988). The Barthel ADL Index: a reliability study. *International Disability Studies*, 10: 61–63.

Conner, K.A., Powers, E. and Bultena, G.L. (1979). 'Social interaction and life satisfaction: an empirical assessment of late life patterns.' *Journal of Gerontology*, 34: 116–21.

Convery, F.R., Minteer, M.A., Amiel, D. and Connett, K.L. (1977). 'Poly-articular disability: a functional assessment.' *Archives of Physical Medicine and Rehabilitation*, 58: 494–9.

Cooper, P.J. and Fairburn, C.G. (1986). 'The depressive symptoms of bulimia nervosa.' *British Journal of Psychiatry*, 148: 268–74.

Coopersmith, S. (1967). *The Antecedents of Self-esteem*. San Francisco, W.H. Freeman. Reprinted in 1981.

Copeland, J.R.M. (1990). 'Suitable instruments for detecting dementia in community samples.' *Age and Ageing*, 19: 81–3.

Copeland, J.R.M. and Gurland, B.J. (1978). 'Evaluation of diagnostic methods: an international comparison' in Isaacs, A.D. and Post, F. (eds). *Studies in Geriatric Psychiatry*. Chichester, John Wiley.

Copeland, J.R.M., Dewey, M.E. and Griffiths Jones, H.M. (1986). 'A computerized psychiatric diagnostic system and case nomenclature for elderly subjects: GMS and AGECAT.' *Psychological Medicine*, 16: 89–99.

Copeland, J.R.M., Dewey, M.E., Wood, N. *et al.* (1987a). 'Range of mental illness among the elderly in the community: prevalence in Liverpool using the GMS-AGECAT package.' *British Journal of Psychiatry*, 150: 815–23.

Copeland, J.R.M., Gurland, B.J., Dewey, M.E. *et al.* (1987b). 'The distribution of dementia, depression and neurosis in elderly men and women in an urban community: assessed using the GMS-AGECAT package.' *International Journal of Geriatric Psychiatry*, 2: 177–84.

Copeland, J.R.M., Dewey, M.E., Henderson, A.S. *et al.* (1988). 'The Geriatric Mental State (GMS) used in the community: replication studies of the computerized diagnoses AGECAT.' *Psychological Medicine*, 18: 219–23.

Copeland, J.R.M., Kelleher, M.J., Kellet, J.M., *et al.* (1976). 'A semi-structured clinical interview for the assessment of diagnosis and mental state in the elderly: The Geriatric Mental State: Schedule I. Development and reliability.' *Psychological Medicine*, 6: 439–49.

Cornoni-Huntley, J.C., Foley, D.J., White, L.R. *et al.* (1985). 'Epidemiology of disability in the oldest old: methodologic issues and preliminary findings.' *Milbank Memorial Fund Quarterly, Health and Society*, 63: 350–76.

Crandall, R.C. (1973). 'The measurement of self esteem and related constructs' in Robinson, J. and Shaver, P. (eds). *Measures of Social Psychological Attitudes.* Ann Arbor, Michigan, Institute for Social Research.

Craven, P. and Wellman, B. (1974). 'The network city' in Effrat, M.P. (ed.). *The Community: Approaches and Applications.* New York, Free Press.

Davidson, I.A., Dewey, M. and Copeland, J.R.M. (1988). 'The relationship between mortality and mental disorder: evidence from the Liverpool longitudinal study.' *International Journal of Geriatric Psychiatry*, 3: 95–8.

Davies, A.R. and Ware, J.E. (1981). *Measuring Health Perceptions in the Health Insurance Program.* Santa Monica, California, Rand Corporation: R-2711–HHS.

Dewey, M.E. and Copeland, J.R.M. (1986). 'Computerized psychiatric diagnosis in the elderly: AGECAT.' *Journal of Microcomputer Applications*, 9: 135–40.

Deyo, R.A., Inui, T.S., Leininger, J.D. *et al.* (1982). 'Physical and psychological functions in rheumatoid arthritis: clinical use of a self-administered instrument.' *Archives of Internal Medicine*, 142: 879–82.

—— (1983). 'Measuring functional outcomes in chronic disease: a comparison of traditional scales and a self-administered health status questionnaire in patients with rheumatoid arthritis.' *Medical Care*, 21: 180–92.

Dobson, C., Powers, E.A., Keith, P.M. *et al.* (1979). 'Anomie, self-esteem, and life satisfaction: interrelationships among three scales of well-being.' *Journal of Gerontology*, 34: 569–72.

Donald, C.A. and Ware, J.E. (1982). *The Quantification of Social Contacts and Resources.* Santa Monica, California, Rand Corporation: R-2937-HHS.

Donald, C.A., Ware, J.E., Brook, R.H. *et al.* (1978). *Conceptualization and measurement of health for adults in the health insurance study*, vol. IV, Social Health. Rand Corporation: Santa Monica, California, R-1987/4-HEW.

Dorn, H.F. (1955). 'Some applications of biometry in the collection and evaluation of medical data.' *Journal of Chronic Diseases*, 1: 638–64.

Dubuisson, D. and Melzack, R. (1976). 'Classification of clinical pain descriptions by multiple group discriminant analysis.' *Experimental Neurology*, 51: 480–7.

Dunnell, K. and Cartwright, A. (1972). *Medicine Takers, Hoarders and Prescribers.* London, Routledge and Kegan Paul.

Dupuy, H.J. (1978). 'Self representations of general psychological well-being of American adults,' paper presented at American Public Health Association Meeting. Los Angeles, California, 17 October.

—— (1984). 'The psychological General Well-being Index' in Wenger, N.K., Mattson, M.E., Furberg, C.D., et al. (eds). Assessment of Quality of Life in Clinical Trials of Cardiovascular Therapies. New York, Le Jacq Publ. Co. Inc.

Ebmeier, K.P., Beson, J.A.O., Eagles, J.N. et al. (1988). 'Continuing care of the demented elderly in Inverurie.' Health Bulletin, 46: 32–41.

Edwards, D.W., Yarvis, R.M., Mueller, D.P. et al. (1978). 'Test-taking and the stability of adjustment scales: can we assess patient deterioration?' Evaluation Q, 2: 275–91.

Edwards, J.N. and Klemmack, D.L. (1973). 'Correlates of life satisfaction: a re-examination.' Journal of Gerontology, 28: 479–502.

Evans, G., Hughes, B.C. and Wilkin, D. (1981). The Management of Mental and Physical Impairment in Non-specialist Residential Homes for the Elderly, Research Report no. 4. Manchester, Research Section, Psychiatric Unit, University Hospital of South Manchester.

Evans, R.W., Manninen, D.L., Overcast, T.D. et al. (1984). The National Heart Transplantation Study: Final Report. Seattle, Washington, Battelle Human Affairs Research Centre.

Fanshel, S. and Bush, J.W. (1970). 'A health status index and its applications to health services outcomes.' Operational Research, 18: 1021–65.

Fazio, A.F. (1977). A Concurrent Validation Study of the NCHS General Well-Being Schedule. Hyattsville, Maryland, US Department of Health, Education and Welfare, National Center for Health Statistics: Vital and Health Statistics Series 2, no. 73 DHEW Publication No. (HRA) 78-1347.

Fillenbaum, G.G. (1978). Validity and Reliability of the Multidimensional Functional Assessment Questionnaire. Multidimensional functional assessment: the OARS Methodology. Duke University, Center for the Study of Aging and Human Development.

Fillenbaum, G.G. and Smyer, M.A. (1981). 'The development, validity and reliability of the OARS multidimensional functional assessment questionnaire: disability and pain scales.' Journal of Gerontology, 36: 428–33.

Finlay-Jones, R.A. and Murphy, E. (1979). 'Severity of psychiatric disorder and the 30-item General Health Questionnaire.' British Journal of Psychiatry, 134: 609–16.

Fiore, J., Coppel, D.B., Becker, J. et al. (1986). 'Social support as a multifaceted concept: examination of important dimensions for adjustment.' American Journal of Community Psychology, 14: 93–111.

Fitts, W.H. (1965). Tennessee Self-Concept Scale Manual. Nashville, Counselor Recordings and Tests.

—— (1972). The Self-Concept and Performance, Research Monograph no. 5. Nashville, Social and Rehabilitation Service.

Fitzpatrick, R., Newman, S., Lamb, R. and Shipley, M. (1989). 'A comparison of measures of health status in rheumatoid arthritis.' British Journal of Rheumatology, 28: 201–6.

Fletcher, A., McLoone, P. and Bulpitt, C. (1988). 'Quality of life on angina therapy: a randomized controlled trial of transdermal glyceryl trinitrate against placebo.' *Lancet*, 2: 4–8.

Fortinsky, R.H., Granger, C.V. and Selzer, G.B. (1981). 'The use of functional assessment in understanding home care needs.' *Medical Care*, 19: 489–97.

Francis, D. (1984). *Will You Still Need Me, Will You Still Feed Me, When I'm 84?* Bloomington, Indiana University Press.

Fries, J.F. (1983). 'The assessment of disability: from first to future principles', paper presented at conference Advances in Assessing Arthritis held at the London Hospital, March (mimeo).

Fries, J.F., Hess, E.V. and Klinenberg, J. (1974). 'A standard database for rheumatic disease.' *Arthritis and Rheumatism*, 17: 327–36.

Fries, J.F., Spitz, P.W., Kraines, R.G. and Holman, H.R. (1980). 'Measurement of patient outcome in arthritis.' *Arthritis and Rheumatism*, 23: 137–45.

Fries, J.F., Spitz, P.W. and Young, D.Y. (1982). 'The dimensions of health outcomes: the Health Assessment Questionnaire, disability and pain scales.' *Journal of Rheumatology*, 9: 789–93.

Gallagher, D., Nies, G. and Thompson, L.W. (1982). 'Reliability of the Beck Depression Inventory with older adults.' *Journal of Consulting and Clinical Psychology*, 50: 152–3.

Gatz, M., Pederson, N.L. and Harris, J. (1987). 'Measurement characteristics of the mental health scale from the OARS.' *Journal of Gerontology*, 42: 332–5.

George, L.K. (1979). 'The happiness syndrome: methodological and substantive issues in the study of psychological well-being in adulthood.' *Gerontologist*, 19: 210–16.

George, L.K. and Bearon, L.B. (1980). *Quality of Life in Older Persons: Meaning and Measurement*. New York, Human Sciences Press.

George, L.K., Blazer, D.G., Hughes, D.C. *et al.* (1989). 'Social support and the outcome of major depression.' *British Journal of Psychiatry*, 154: 478–85.

Gilson, B.S., Bergner, M., Bobbitt, R.A. *et al.* (1979). *The Sickness Impact Profile: Final Development and Testing: 1975–1978*. Seattle, University of Washington Press.

Goldberg, D.P. (1978). *Manual of the General Health Questionnaire*. Windsor, NFER-Nelson.

—— (1985). 'Identifying psychiatric illness among general medical patients.' *British Medical Journal*, 291: 161–3.

Goldberg, D.P. and Huxley, P. (1980). *Mental Illness in the Community: The Pathway to Psychiatric Care*. London, Tavistock.

Goldberg, D.P. and Williams, P. (1988). *A user's guide to the General Health Questionnaire*. Windsor, NFER-Nelson.

Goldberg, E.M. and Connelly, N. (1982). *The Effectiveness of Social Care for the Elderly*. London, Heinemann.

Goldstein, M.S., Siegel, J.M. and Boyer, R. (1984). 'Predicting changes in perceived health status.' *American Journal of Public Health*, 74: 611–15.

Goodchild, M.E. and Duncan Jones, P. (1985). 'Chronicity and the General Health Questionnaire.' *British Journal of Psychiatry*, 146: 55–61.

Gough, I.R., Furnival, C.M., Schilder, L. *et al.* (1983). 'Assessment of the quality of life of patients with advanced cancer.' *European Journal of Cancer and Clinical Oncology*, 19: 1161–5.

Graham, C., Bond, S.S., Gerkovich, M.M. *et al.* (1980). 'Use of the McGill pain questionnaire in the assessment of cancer pain: reliability and consistency.' *Pain*, 6: 377.

Granger, C.V. and McNamara, M.A. (1984). 'Functional assessment utilization: the long-range evaluation system (LRES)' in Granger, C.V. and Gresham, G.E. (eds). *Functional Assessment in Rehabilitation Medicine*. Baltimore, Williams & Williams.

Granger, C.V., Albrecht, G.L. and Hamilton, B.B. (1979). 'Outcome of comprehensive medical rehabilitation: measurement by PULSES profile and the Barthel Index.' *Archives of Physical Medicine and Rehabilitation*, 60: 145–54.

Grant, C.R.H. (1966). 'Age differences in self-concept from early adulthood through old age.' Dissertation from the University of Nebraska.

Grasbeck, R. and Saris, N.E. (1969). 'Establishment and use of normal values.' *Scandinavian Journal of Clinical and Laboratory Investigation*, Supplement no. 110: 62–3.

Greenblatt, H.N. (1975). *Measurement of Social Well-being in a General Population Survey*. Berkeley, Human Population Laboratory, California State Department of Health.

Greenblatt, M.Y., Becerra, R.M. and Serafetinides, E.A. (1982). 'Social networks and mental health: an overview.' *American Journal of Psychiatry*, 139: 977–84.

Greenwald, H.P. (1987). 'The specificity of quality of life measures among the seriously ill.' *Medical Care*, 25: 642–51.

Gurin, G., Veroff, J. and Feld, S. (1960). *Americans View their Mental Health*. New York, Basic Books.

Gurland, B.J. (1980). 'The assessment of the mental health status of older adults' in Birren, J.E. and Sloane, R.B. (eds). *Handbook of Mental Health and Ageing*. Englewood Cliffs, NJ, Prentice-Hall.

Gurland, B.J., Copeland, J.R.M., Kelleher, M.J. *et al.* (1983). *The Mind and Mood of Ageing: The Mental Health Problems of the Community Elderly in New York and London*. London, Croom Helm.

Guttman, L. (1944). 'A basis for scaling qualitative data.' *American Sociological Review*, 9: 139.

Haber, L.D. (1968). *Prevalence of Disability among Non-institutionalized Adults under Age 65: 1966 Survey of Disabled Adults*, Research and Statistics Note no. 4. US Department of Health Education and Welfare, Office of Research and Statistics.

Hall, J., Hall, N., Fisher, E. *et al.* (1987). 'Measurement of outcomes of general practice: comparison of three health status measures.' *Family Practice*, 4: 117–23.

Hall, R., Horrocks, J.C., Clamp, S.E. *et al.* (1976). 'Observer variation in assessment of results of surgery for peptic ulceration.' *British Medical Journal*, i: 814–16.

Hamilton, M. (1959). 'The assessment of anxiety states by rating.' *British Journal of Medical Psychology*, 32: 50–5.

—— (1967). 'Development of a rating scale for primary depressive illness.' *British Journal of Social and Clinical Psychology*, 6: 278–96.

—— (1976). 'Clinical evaluation of depression: clinical criteria and rating scales, including a Guttman Scale' in Gallant, D.M. and Simpson, G.M. (eds).

Depression: Behavioral, Biochemical Diagnostic and Treatment Concepts. New York, Spectrum Publications.

Hammen, C.L. (1981). 'Assessment: a clinical and cognitive emphasis' in Rehm, L.P. (ed.). *Behaviour Therapy for Depression: Present Status and Future Directions*. New York, Academic Press.

Harman, H.H. (1976). *Modern Factor Analysis*. Chicago, University of Chicago Press.

Harris, L. (1975). *The Myth and Reality of Ageing in America*. Washington, D.C., National Council on the Ageing.

Hart, G.L. and Evans, R.W. (1987). 'The functional status of ESRD patients as measured by the Sickness Impact Profile.' *Journal of Chronic Diseases*, 40: 117S–130S (Supplement).

Heasman, M.A. and Lipworth, L. (1966). *Accuracy of Certification of Cause of Death*. London, General Register Office. Studies on Medical and Population Subjects no. 20.

Henderson, A.S., Duncan Jones, P. and Finlay-Jones, R.A. (1983). 'The reliability of the Geriatric Mental State Examination.' *Acta Psychiatrica Scandinavica*, 67: 281–9.

Henderson, S. (1981). 'Social relationships, adversity and neurosis: an analysis of prospective observations.' *British Journal of Psychiatry*, 138: 391–8.

Henderson, S., Byrne, D.G. and Duncan Jones, P. (1981a). *Neurosis and the Social Environment*. London, Academic Press.

Henderson, S., Duncan Jones, P., Byrne, D.G., *et al.* (1980). 'Measuring social relationships: the Interview Schedule for Social Interaction.' *Psychological Medicine*, 10: 723–34.

Henderson, S., Lewis, I.C., Howell, R.H. *et al.* (1981b). 'Mental health and the use of alcohol, tobacco, analgesics and vitamins in a secondary school population.' *Acta Psychiatrica Scandinavica*, 63: 186–9.

Herron, M.K., Michaux, W.W., Katz, M.M. *et al.* (1964). *Supplemental Instructions for the Administration of the Katz Adjustment Scales*. Baltimore, Spring Grove State Hospital, Research Department.

Hinterberger, W., Gadner, H., Hocker, P. *et al.* (1987). 'Survival and quality of life in 23 patients with severe aplastic anaemia treated with BMT.' *Blut*, 54: 137–46.

Hirsch, B.J. (1980). 'Natural support systems and coping with major life changes.' *American Journal of Community Psychology*, 8: 159–72.

—— (1981). 'Social networks and the coping process: creating personal communities' in Gottlieb, B.H. (ed.). *Social Networks and Social Support*. Beverly Hills, Sage Publications.

Hobbs, P., Ballinger, C.B., Greenwood, C. *et al.* (1984). 'Factor analysis and validation of the General Health Questionnaire in men: a general practice survey.' *British Journal of Psychiatry*, 144: 270–5.

Hobbs, P., Ballinger, C.B. and Smith, A.H.W. (1983). 'Factor analysis and validation of the General Health Questionnaire in women: a general practice survey.' *British Journal of Psychiatry*, 142: 257–64.

Hodkinson, H.M. (1972). 'Evaluation of a mental test score for the assessment of mental impairment in the elderly.' *Age and Ageing*, 1: 233–8.

Hoffmeister, J.K. (1976). *Some Information Regarding the Characteristics of the Two*

Measures Developed from the Self-Esteem Questionnaire (SEQ-3). Boulder, CO, Test Analysis and Development Corporation.

Holahan, C.J. and Moos, R.H. (1981). 'Social support and psychological distress: a longitudinal analysis'. *Journal of Abnormal Psychology*, 90: 365–70.

House, J.S. (1981). *Work, Stress and Social Support.* Reading, Massachusetts, Addison-Wesley.

House, J.S. and Kahn, R.L. (1985). 'Measures and concepts of social support' in Cohen, S. and Syme, S.L. (eds). *Social Support and Health.* Orlando, Academic Press.

House, J.S., Robbins, C. and Metzner, H.L. (1982). 'The association of social relationships and activities with mortality: prospective evidence from the Tecumseh Community Health Study.' *American Journal of Epidemiology*, 116: 123–40.

Hoyt, D.R. and Creech, J.C. (1983). 'The life satisfaction index: a methodological and theoretical critique.' *Journal of Gerontology*, 38: 111–16.

Hoyt, D.R., Kaiser, M., Peters, G. *et al.* (1980). 'Life satisfaction and activity theory: a multidimensional approach.' *Journal of Gerontology*, 35: 935–41.

Hunt, S.M. (1986). 'Measuring health in clinical care and clinical trials' in Teeling Smith G. (ed.). *Measuring health: a practical approach.* Chichester, John Wiley.

—— (1988). 'Subjective health indicators and health promotion.' *Health Promotion*, 3: 23–34.

Hunt, S.M., McEwan, J. and McKenna, S.P. (1984). 'Perceived health: age and sex comparisons in a community.' *Journal of Epidemiology and Community Health*, 34: 281–6.

—— (1986). *Measuring Health Status.* London, Croom Helm.

Hunt, S.M., McKenna, S.P., McEwan, J. *et al.* (1980). 'A quantitative approach to perceived health status: a validation study.' *Journal of Epidemiology and Community Health*, 34: 281–6.

Hunt, S.M., McKenna, S.P. and Williams, J. (1981). 'Reliability of a population survey tool for measuring perceived health problems: a study of patients with osteo-arthritis.' *Journal of Epidemiology and Community Health*, 35: 297–300.

Hutchinson, T.A., Boyd, N.F. and Feinstein, A.R. (1979). 'Scientific problems in clinical scales as demonstrated in the Karnofsky index of performance status.' *Journal of Chronic Diseases*, 32: 661–6.

Isaacs, B. and Walkey, P.A. (1964). 'Measurement of mental impairment in geriatric pratice.' *Gerontology Clinics*, 6: 114–23.

Jachuck, S.J., Brierly, H., Jachuk, S. *et al.* (1982). 'The effect of hypotensive drugs on the quality of life.' *Journal of the Royal College of General Practitioners*, 32: 103–5.

Jenkinson, C., Fitzpatrick, R. and Argyle, M. (1988). 'The Nottingham Health Profile: an analysis of its sensitivity in differentiating illness groups.' *Social Science and Medicine*, 27: 1411–14.

Jitapunkul, S., Pillay, I. and Ebrahim, S. (1991). The Abbreviated Mental Test: its use and validity. *Age and Ageing*, 20: 332–336.

Jones, D.A., Victor, C.R. and Vetter, N.J. (1985). 'The problem of loneliness in the elderly in the community: characteristics of those who are lonely and the factors related to the loneliness.' *Journal of the Royal College of General Practitioners*, 35: 136–9.

Kahn, R.L., Goldfarb, A.I., Pollack, M. *et al.* (1960a). 'The relationship of mental and physical status in institutionalized aged persons.' *American Journal of Psychiatry*, 117: 120–4.

—— (1960b). 'Brief objective measures for the determination of mental status in the aged.' *American Journal of Psychiatry*, 117: 326–8.

Kalson, C. (1976). 'MASH – a program of social interaction between institutionalised aged and adult mentally retarded persons.' *The Gerontologist*, 16: 340–8.

Kammann, R. and Flett, R. (1983). 'Affectometer 2: a scale to measure current level of general happiness.' *Australian Journal of Psychology*, 35: 259–65.

Kaplan, B.H. (1975). 'An epilogue: toward further research on family and health' in Kaplan, B.H. and Cassel, J.C. (eds). *Family and Health: An Epidemiological Approach*. University of North Carolina, Institute for Research and Social Science, Chapel Hill.

Kaplan, G.A. and Camacho, T. (1983). 'Perceived health and mortality: a nine-year follow-up of the Human Population Laboratory Cohort.' *American Journal of Epidemiology*, 117: 292–8.

Kaplan, H.B. and Porkorny, A.D. (1969). 'Self derogation and psychosocial adjustment.' *Journal of Nervous and Mental Disease*, 149: 421–34.

Kaplan, R. (1985). 'Social support and social health' in Saranson, I. and Saranson, B. (eds). *Social Support Theory, Research and Application*. The Hague, Nijhoff.

Kaplan, R.M. (1988). 'New health promotion indicators: the general health policy model.' *Health Promotion*, 3: 35–48.

Kaplan, R.M. and Bush, J.W. (1982). 'Health-related quality of life measurement for evaluation research analysis.' *Health Psychology*, 1: 61–80.

Kaplan, R.M. and Ernst, J.A. (1983). 'Do category rating scales produce biased preference weights for a health index?' *Medical Care*, 21: 193–207.

Kaplan, R.M., Bush, J.W. and Berry, C.C. (1976). 'Health status: types of validity and the Index of Well-being.' *Health Services Research*, 11: 478–507.

—— (1978). 'The reliability, stability and generalizability of a health status index.' American Statistical Association, Proceedings of the Social Statistics Section: 704–9.

—— (1979). 'Health Status Index: category rating versus magnitude estimation for measuring levels of well-being.' *Medical Care*, 17: 501–23.

Karnofsky, D.A., Abelmann, W.H., Craver, L.F. *et al.* (1948). 'The use of nitrogen mustards in the palliative treatment of carcinoma.' *Cancer*, I: 634–56.

Kasl, S.V. and Cooper, C.L. (1987). *Stress and Health Issues in Research Methodology*. Chichester, John Wiley.

Katz, S. and Akpom, C.A. (1976). 'Index of ADL.' *Medical Care*, 14: 116–18.

Katz, S., Akpom, C.A., Papsidero, J.A. *et al.* (1973). 'Measuring the health status of populations' in Berg, R.L. (ed.). *Health Status of Populations*. Chicago, Hospital Research and Educational Trust.

Katz, S., Downs, T.D., Cash, H.R. *et al.* (1970). 'Progress in the development of and index of ADL.' *Gerontologist*, 10: 20–30.

Katz, S., Ford, A.B., Chinn, A.B. *et al.* (1966). 'Prognosis after strokes: long-term course of 159 patients.' *Medicine*, 45: 236.

Katz, S., Ford, A.B., Moskowitz, R.W. *et al.* (1963). 'Studies of illness in the aged: the index of ADL – a standardized measure of biological and psychosocial function.' *Journal of the American Medical Association*, 185: 914–19.

Katz, S., Vignos, P.J., Moskowitz, R.W. *et al.* (1968). 'Comprehensive outpatient care in rheumatoid arthritis: a controlled study.' *Journal of the American Medicine Association*, 206: 1249.

Kay, D.W.K., Beamish, R. and Roth, M. (1964). 'Old age mental disorders in Newcastle upon Tyne, Part I: a study of prevalence.' *British Journal of Psychiatry*, 110: 146–58.

Kazis, L.E., Anderson, J.J. and Meenan, R.F. (1988). 'Health status information in clinical practice: the development and testing of patient profile reports.' *Journal of Rheumatology*, 15: 338–44.

Kazis, L.E., Meenan, R.F. and Anderson, J.J. (1983). 'Pain in the rheumatic diseases: investigation of a key health status component.' *Arthritis and Rheumatism*, 26: 1017–22.

Kelley, T.L. (1927). *Interpretation of Educational Measurements*. Yonkers, World Books.

Kind, P. (undated). 'Scaling the Nottingham Health Profile.' Mimeo, University of York, York, Centre for Health Economics.

Kind, P. and Carr-Hill, R. (1987). 'The Nottingham Health Profile: a useful tool for epidemiologists?' *Social Science and Medicine*, 25: 905–10.

Kirwan, R.J. and Reeback, J.S. (1983). 'Using a modified Stanford Health Assessment Questionnaire to assess disability in UK patients with rheumatoid arthritis.' *Annals of the Rheumatic Diseases*, 42: 219–20.

Knapp, M.R.J. (1976). 'Predicting the dimensions of life satisfaction.' *Journal of Gerontology*, 31: 595–604.

Kohn, M.L. (1969). *Class and Conformity: a Study in Values*. Homewood, Illinois, Dorsey.

Kokenes, B. (1974). 'Grade level differences in factors of self esteem.' *Development Psychology*, 10: 954–8.

Kozma, A. and Stones, M.J. (1987). 'Social desirability in measures of subjective well-being: a systematic evaluation.' *Journal of Gerontology*, 42: 56–9.

Kushman, J. and Lane, S. (1980). 'A multivariate analysis of factors affecting perceived life satisfaction and psychological well-being among the elderly.' *Social Science Quarterly*, 61: 264–77.

Kutner, B., Fansel, D., Togo, A.M. *et al.* (1956). *Five Hundred over 60*. New York, Russell Sage.

Kutner, N.G., Fair, P.L. and Kutner, M.H. (1985). 'Assessing depression and anxiety in chronic dialysis patients.' *Journal of Psychosomatic Research*, 29: 23–31.

Lamb, K.L., Brodie, D.A. and Roberts, K. (1988). 'Physical fitness and health-related fitness as indicators of a positive health state.' *Health Promotion*, 3: 171–82.

Larson, R. (1978). 'Thirty years of research on the subjective well-being of older Americans.' *Journal of Gerontology*, 33: 109–25.

Lawton, M.P. (1972). 'The dimensions of morale' in Kent, D., Kastenbaum, R. and Sherwood, S. (eds). *Research, Planning and Action for the Elderly*. New York, Behavioral Publications.

—— (1975). 'The Philadelphia Geriatric Center Morale Scale: a revision.' *Journal of Gerontology*, 30: 85–9.

Leighton, A.H. (1959). *My Name is Legion: Foundations for a Theory of Man in Relation to Culture.* New York, Basic Books.

Leighton Read, J., Quinn, R.J. and Hoefer, M.A. (1987). 'Measuring overall health: an evaluation of three important approaches.' *Journal of Chronic Diseases*, 40: Supplement 1: 7S–21S.

Lerner, M. (1973). 'Conceptualization of health and well-being.' *Health Services Research*, 8: 6–12.

Liang, J. (1984). 'Dimensions of the life satisfaction Index A: a structural formation.' *Journal of Gerontology*, 39: 613–22.

Liang, J. and Bollen, K.A. (1983). 'The structure of the Philadelphia Center Morale Scale: a reinterpretation.' *Journal of Gerontology*, 30: 77–84.

Liem, G.R. and Liem, J.H. (1978). *Social support and stress. Some general issues and their application to the problems of unemployment.* Unpublished manuscript. Boston College and University of Massachusetts.

Likert, R. (1952). 'A technique for the development of attitude scales.' *Educational and Psychological Measurement*, 12: 313–15.

Lin, N., Simeone, R., Ensel, W. *et al.* (1979). 'Social support, stressful life events and illness, a model and an empirical test.' *Journal of Health and Social Behaviour*, 20: 108–19.

Lohmann, N. (1977). 'Correlations of life satisfaction, morale and adjustment measures.' *Journal of Gerontology*, 32: 73–5.

Lowe, D.J. (1975). *The Cornell Indices: A Bibliography of Health Questionnaires.* Cornell University Medical College Library, Reference and Information Services, New York.

Lowenthal, M.F. and Haven, C. (1968). 'Interaction and adaptation: intimacy as a critical variable.' *American Sociological Review*, 33: 20–30.

McDowell, I. and Newell, C. (1987). *Measuring Health: A Guide to Rating Scales and Questionnaires.* New York, Oxford University Press.

McFarlane, A.H., Neale, K.A., Norman, G. *et al.* (1981). 'Methodological issues in developing a scale to measure social support.' *Schizophrenia Bulletin*, 7: 90–100.

McKenna, S.P., Hunt, S.M. and McEwan, J. (1981). 'Weighting the seriousness of perceived health problems using Thurstone's method of paired comparisons.' *International Journal of Epidemiology*, 10: 93–7.

McKenna, S.P., McEwan, J., Hunt, S.M. *et al.* (1984). 'Changes in the perceived health of patients recovering from fractures.' *Public Health*, 98: 97–102.

McKennell, A.C. (1978). 'Cognitive and affect in perceptions of well-being.' *Social Indicators Research*, 5: 389–426.

McNab, A. and Phillip, A.S. (1980). 'Screening an elderly population for psychological well-being.' *Health Bulletin*, 160–5.

McNeil, B.J., Weichselbaum, R. and Pauker, S.G. (1978). 'Fallacy of the five year survival in lung cancer.' *New England Journal of Medicine*, 299: 1397–401.

—— (1981). 'Speech and Survival: tradeoffs between quality and quantity of life in laryngeal cancer.' *New England Journal of Medicine*, 305: 982–7.

McPeek, B. and McPeek, A. (1984). 'Formen der Wiedergabe der Lebensqualitat in Klinischen Studien' in Rohde, H. and Troidl, Hans (eds). *Das Magenkarzinom:*

Methodik Klinischer Studien und therapeutischer Ansatze. New York, Georg Thieme Verlag.

McWilliam, C., Copeland, J.R.M., Dewey, M.E. *et al.* (1988). 'The geriatric mental state examination as a case finding instrument in the community.' *British Journal of Psychiatry*, 152: 205–8.

Maes, S., Vingerhoets, A. and Van Heck, G. (1987). 'The study of stress and disease: some developments and requirements.' *Social Science and Medicine*, 25: 567–78.

Mahoney, F.I. and Barthel, D.W. (1965). 'Functional evaluation: the Barthel Index.' *Maryland State Medical Journal*, 14: 61–5.

Mari, J.D.J. and Williams, P. (1985). 'A comparison of the validity of two psychiatric screening questionnaires (GHQ-12 and SRQ-20) in Brazil, using relative operating characteristics (ROC) analysis.' *Psychological Medicine*, 15: 651–9.

Martin, A.J. (1987). 'Patients and presentation: a profile from general practice.' *Modern Medicine*, April: 14–18.

Mason, J.H., Anderson, J.J. and Meenan, R.F. (1988). 'A model for health status for rheumatoid arthritis: a factor analysis of the Arthritis Impact Measurement Scales.' *Arthritis and Rheumatism*, 31: 714–20.

Meenan, R.F. (1982). 'The AIMS approach to health status measurement: conceptual background and measurement properties.' *Journal of Rheumatology*, 9: 785–8.

—— (1985). 'New approaches to outcome assessment: the AIMS questionnaire for arthritis' in Stollerman, G.H. (ed.). *Advances in Internal Medicine*, vol. 31. New York, Year Book Medical Publishers.

Meenan, R.F., Anderson, J.J., Kazis, L.E. *et al.* (1984). 'Outcome assessment in clinical trials: evidence for the sensitivity of a health status measure.' *Arthritis and Rheumatism*, 27: 1344–52.

Meenan, R.F., Gertman, P.M. and Mason, J.H. (1980). 'Measuring health status in arthritis: the arthritis impact measurement scales.' *Arthritis and Rheumatism*, 23: 146–52.

Meenan, R.F., Gertman, P.M., Mason, J.H. *et al.* (1982). 'The arthritis impact measurement scales: further investigations of a health status measure.' *Arthritis and Rheumatism*, 25: 1048–53.

Mellor, K.S. and Edelmann, R.J. (1988). 'Mobility, social support, loneliness and well-being amongst two groups of older adults.' *Journal of Personality and Individual Differences*, 9: 1–5.

Melzack, R. (1975). 'The McGill pain questionnaire: major properties and scoring methods.' *Pain*, 1: 277.

—— (1983). Pain measurement and assessment. New York, Raven Press.

—— (1987). 'The short-form McGill Pain Questionnaire.' *Pain*, 30: 191–7.

Melzack, R. and Torgerson, W.S. (1971). 'On the language of pain.' *Anesthesiology*, 34: 50.

Mendola, W.F. and Pelligrini, R.V. (1979). 'Quality of life and coronary artery bypass surgery patients.' *Social Science and Medicine*, 13A, 457–61.

Merrell, M. and Harris, L. (1975). *The Myth and Reality of Ageing in America.* Washington, DC, National Council on Ageing.

Merrell, M. and Reed, L.J. (1949). *The epidemiology of health, social medicine, its deviations and objectives*. New York, The Commonwealth Fund.

Messick, S. (1980). 'Test validity and the ethics of assessment.' *American Psychologist*, 35: 1012–27.

Milne, J.S., Maule, M.M., Cormack, S. *et al.* (1972). 'The design and testing of a questionnaire and examination to assess physical and mental health in older people using a staff nurse as the observer.' *Journal of Chronic Diseases*, 25: 385–405.

Mitchell, J.C. (1969). 'The concept and use of social networks' in Mitchell, J.C. (ed.). *Social Networks in Urban Situations: Analysis of Personal Relationships in Central African Towns*. Manchester, Manchester University Press.

Mitchell, R.E. and Trickett, E.J. (1980). 'Social networks as mediators of social support: an analysis of the effects and determinants ot social networks.' *Community Mental Health Journal*, 16: 27–44.

Monk, M. (1981). 'Blood pressure awareness and psychological well-being in the Health and Nutrition Examination Survey.' *Clinical Investigative Medicine*, 4: 183–9.

Montgomery, S.A. and Asberg, M. (1979). 'A new depression scale designed to be sensitive to change.' *British Journal of Psychiatry*, 134: 382–9.

Moos, R.H. and Moos, B.S. (1981). *Manual for Family Environment Scale*. Palo Alto, CA, Consulting Psychologists Press.

Mor, V. (1987). 'Cancer patients' quality of life over the disease course: lessons from the real world.' *Journal of Chronic Disease*, 40: 535–44.

Mor, V., Laliberte, L., Morris, J.N. *et al.* (1984). 'The Karnofsky performance status scale: an examination of its reliability and validity in a research setting.' *Cancer*, 53: 2002–7.

Morgan, K., Dallosso, H.M., Arie, T. *et al.* (1987). 'Mental health and psychological well-being among the old and the very old living at home.' *British Journal of Psychiatry*, 150: 801–7.

Moriyama, I.M. (1968). 'Problems in the measurement of health status' in Sheldon, E.B. and Moore, W.E. (eds). *Indicators of Social Change*. New York, Russell Sage Foundation.

Morris, J. (1975). 'Changes in morale experienced by the elderly institutionalized applicants along the institutional path.' *Gerontologist*, 15: 345–9.

Morris, J.N. and Sherwood, S. (1975). 'A re-testing and modification of the Philadelphia Geriatric Center Morale Scale.' *Journal of Gerontology*, 30: 77–84.

—— (1987). 'Quality of life of cancer patients at different stages in the disease trajectory.' *Journal of Chronic Disease*, 40: 545–53.

Morris, J., Suissa, A., Sherwood, S. *et al.* (1986). 'Last days: a study of the quality of life of terminally ill cancer patients.' *Journal of Chronic Disease*, 39: 47–62.

Morris, L.W., Morris, R.G. and Britton, P.G. (1989). 'Social support networks and formal support as factors influencing the psychological adjustment of spouse caregivers of dementia sufferers.' *International Journal of Geriatric Psychiatry*, 4: 47–51.

Morton-Williams, J. (1979). 'Alternative patterns of care for the elderly: Methodological report.' *Social and Community Planning Research*. London.

Mulgrave, N.W. (1985). 'Clifton Assessment Procedures for the elderly' in

Keyser, D.J. and Sweetland, R.C. (eds). *Test Critiques*, vol. II. Kansas City, Missouri.

National Center for Health Statistics. *Health Survey Procedures: Concepts, Questionnaires, Development and Definitions in the Health Interview Survey*, Publication no. 1000, Series 1, No. 2, Washington, Public Health Service, May, 1964.

National Heart and Lung Institute (1976). 'Report of a task group on cardiac rehabilitation' in *Proceedings of the Heart and Lung Institute Working Conference on Health Behaviour*. Bethesda, MD, US Department of Health, Education and Welfare.

Neugarten, B.L., Havighurst, R.J. and Tobin, S.S. (1961). 'The measurement of life satisfaction.' *Journal of Gerontology*, 16: 134–43.

Noack, H. and McQueen, D. (1988). 'Towards health promotion indicators.' *Health Promotion*, 3: 73–8.

Noelker, L. and Harel, Z. (1978). 'Predictors of well-being and survival among institutionalized aged.' *Gerontologist*, 18: 562–7.

O'Brien, B.J. (1988). 'Assessment of treatment in heart disease' in Teeling Smith, G. (ed.). *Measuring Health: A Practical Approach*. Chichester, John Wiley.

O'Brien, B.J., Banner, N.R., Gibson, S. *et al.* (1988). 'The Nottingham Health Profile as a measure of quality of life following combined heart and lung transplantation.' *Journal of Epidemiology and Community Health*, 42: 232–4.

Office of Population Censuses and Surveys (1987). *General Household Survey (1985)* London, HMSO.

Olsson, G., Lubsen, J. and Van Es, G.A. (1986). 'Quality of life after myocardial infarction: effect of long-term metoprolol on mortality and morbidity.' *British Medical Journal*, 292: 1491–3.

O'Reilly, P. (1988). 'Methodological issues in social support and social network research.' *Social Science and Medicine*, 26: 863–73.

O'Riordan, T.G., Haynes, J.P. and O'Neil, D. (1990). 'The effect of mild to moderate dementia on the Geriatric Depression Scale and on the General Health Questionnaire.' *Age and Ageing*, 19: 57–61.

Orth-Gomer, K. and Johnson, J. (1987). 'Social network interaction and mortality. A six-year follow-up study of a random sample of the Swedish population.' *Journal of Chronic Diseases*, 40: 949–57.

Orth-Gomer, K. and Unden, A.L. (1987). 'The measurement of social support in population surveys.' *Social Science and Medicine*, 24: 83–94.

Orth-Gomer, K., Britton, M. and Rehnqvist, N. (1979). 'Quality of care in an out-patient department: the patient's view.' *Social Science and Medicine*, 13A: 347–57.

Ott, C.R., Sivarajan, E.S., Newton, K.M. *et al.* (1983). 'A controlled randomized study of early cardiac rehabilitation: the Sickness Impact Profile as an assessment tool.' *Heart and Lung*, 12: 162–70.

Ottawa Charter for Health Promotion (1986). *Health Promotion*, 14: iii–v.

O'Young, J. and McPeek, B. (1987). 'Quality of life variables in surgical trials.' *Journal of Chronic Diseases*, 40: 513–22.

Paterson, M. (1988). 'Treatment in rheumatoid arthritis' in Teeling Smith, G. (ed.). *Measuring Health: A Practical Approach*. Chichester, John Wiley.

Patterson, W. (1975). 'The quality of survival in response to treatment.' *Journal of the American Medical Association*, 233: 280–1.

Patrick, D.L. (ed.). (1982). *Health and Care of the Physically Disabled in Lambeth*. Report of Phase II of the Longitudinal Disability Interview Survey. London, St. Thomas's Hospital Medical School, Department of Community Medicine.

Patrick, D.L., Bush, J.W. and Chen, M.M. (1973a). 'Methods for measuring levels of well-being for a health status index.' *Health Services Research*, 11: 516.

—— (1973b). 'Toward an operational definition of health.' *Journal of Health and Social Behaviour*, 14: 6–23.

Pattie, A.H. and Gilleard, C.J. (1979). *Manual of the Clifton Assessment Procedures for the Elderly*. Sevenoaks, Hodder and Stoughton.

Payne, R.L. and Graham-Jones, J. (1987). 'Measurement and methodological issues in social support' in Kasl, S.V. and Cooper, C.L. (eds). *Stress and Health: Issues in Research Methodology*. Chichester, John Wiley.

Perlman, D. and Peplau, L.A. (1981). 'Toward a social psychology of loneliness' in Gilmour R. and Duck S. (eds). *Personal relationships: 3. Personal relationships in disorder*. London, Academic Press.

Perlman, R.A. (1987). 'Development of a functional assessment questionnaire for geriatric patients: the comprehensive older persons' evaluation (COPE).' *Journal of Chronic Diseases*, 40: 85S–94S, Supplement.

Perloff, J.M. and Persons, J.B. (1988). 'Biases resulting from the use of indexes: an application to attributional style and depression.' *Psychological Bulletin*, 103: 95–104.

Pfeiffer, E. (1975). 'A short portable mental status questionnaire for the assessment of organic brain deficit in elderly patients.' *Journal of American Geriatrics Society*, 23: 433–41.

Pollard, W.E., Bobbitt, R.A. and Bergner, M. (1978). 'Examination of variable errors of measurement in a survey-based social indicator.' *Social Indicators Research*, 5: 279–301.

Pollard, W.E., Bobbitt, R.A., Bergner, M., *et al.* (1976). 'The Sickness Impact Profile: reliability of a health status measure.' *Medical Care*, 14: 57–67.

Priestman, T.J. and Baum, M. (1976). 'Evaluation of quality of life in patients receiving treatment for advanced breast cancer.' *Lancet*, i: 899–901.

Prieto, E.J. and Geisinger, K.F. (1983). 'Factor analytic studies of the McGill Pain Questionnaire' in Melzack, R. (ed.). *Pain Measurement and Assessment*. New York, Raven Press.

Procidano, M.E. and Heller, K. (1983). 'Measures of perceived social support from friends and from family: three validation studies.' *American Journal of Community Psychology*, 11: 1–24.

Qureshi, K.N. and Hodkinson, H.M. (1974). 'Evaluation of a 10 question mental test in the institutionalized elderly.' *Age and Ageing*, 3: 152–7.

Read, L.J., Quinn, R.J. and Hoefer, M.A. (1987). 'Measuring overall health: an evaluation of three important approaches.' *Journal of Chronic Diseases*, 40: 7S–21S.

Reading, A.E. (1979). 'The internal structure of the McGill Pain Questionnaire in dysmenorrhoea patients.' *Pain*, 7: 353–8.

Reed, P.F., Fitts, W.H. and Boehm, L. (1980). *Tennessee Self Concept Scale:*

Bibliography of Research Studies. Nashville, Tennessee, Councillor Recordings and Tests.

Rehm, L.P. (1981). *Behaviour Therapy for Depression.* New York, Academic Press.

Renne, K.S. (1974). 'Measurement of social health in a general population survey.' *Social Sciences Research*, 3: 25–44.

Reynolds, W.M. and Gould, J.W. (1981). 'A psychometric investigation of the standard and short form Beck Depression Inventory.' *Journal of Consulting and Clinical Psychology*, 49: 306–7.

Robinson, J.P. and Shaver, P.R. (1973). *Measures of Social Psychological Attitudes.* Ann Arbor, Mich., Survey Research Centre, Institute for Social Research.

Robinson, R.A. (1968). 'The organisation of a diagnostic and treatment unit for the aged' in Giegy, U.K. *Psychiatric Disorders in the Aged.* Manchester, World Psychiatric Association.

Rosenberg, M. (1965). *Society and the Adolescent Self Image.* Princeton, NJ, Princeton University Press.

Rosser, R.M. and Watts, V.C. (1971). 'The sanative outputs of hospitals.' Dallas, 39th conference of the Operational Research Society of America.

Roth, M., Tym, E., Mountjoy, C.Q. *et al.* (1986). 'CAMDEX: a standardized instrument for the diagnosis of mental disorder in the elderly with special reference to the early detection of dementia.' *British Journal of Psychiatry*, 149: 698–709.

Russell, D. (1982). 'The measurement of loneliness' in Peplau, L.A. and Perlman, D. (eds). *Loneliness: A Sourcebook of Current Theory, Research and Therapy.* New York, John Wiley.

Russell, D., Peplau, L.A. and Cutrona, C.E. (1980). 'The revised UCLA Loneliness Scale: concurrent and discriminant validity evidence.' *Journal of Personality and Social Psychology*, 39: 472–80.

Russell, D., Peplau, L.A. and Ferguson, M.L. (1978). 'Developing a measure of loneliness.' *Journal of Personality Assessment*, 42: 290–4.

Sackett, D.L., Spitzer, W.O., Gent, M. *et al.* (1974). 'The Burlington Randomized Trial of the nurse practitioner: health outcomes of patients. *Annals of Internal Medicine*, 80: 137–42.

Sainsbury, S. (1973). *Measuring Disability.* London, Bell.

Sandler, I.N. and Barrera, M. (1984). 'Towards a multimethod approach to assessing the effects of social support.' *American Journal of Community Psychology*, 12: 37–52.

Sarason, I.G., Levine, H.M., Basham, R.B. *et al.* (1983). 'Assessing social support: the social support questionnaire.' *Journal of Personality and Social Psychology*, 44: 127–39.

Saronson, S.B., Carroll, C., Maton, K. *et al.* (1977). *Human Services and Resource Networks.* San Francisco, Jossey-Bass.

Saunders, P.A., Copeland, J.R., Dewey, M.E. *et al.* (1989). 'Alcohol use and abuse in the elderly: findings from the Liverpool longitudinal study of continuing health in the community.' *International Journal of Geriatric Psychiatry*, 4: 103–8.

Schag, C.C., Heinrich, R.L. and Ganz, P.A. (1983). 'Cancer Inventory of Problem Situations: an instrument for assessing cancer patients' rehabilitation needs.' *Journal of Psychosocial Oncology*, 1: 11–22.

—— (1984). 'Karnofsky performance status revisited, validity and guidelines.' *Journal of Clinical Oncology*, 2: 187–93.

Schwartz, A.N. (1975). 'An observation of self-esteem as the linchpin of quality of life for the aged. An essay.' *Gerontologist*, 15: 470–2.

Scott, P.J., Ansell, B.M. and Huskisson, E.C. (1977). 'The measurement of pain in juvenile chronic polyarthritis.' *Annals of the Rheumatic Diseases*, 36: 186–7.

Scottish Health Education Group (1984). European Monographs in Health Education Research, no. 6. Edinburgh, Scottish Health Education Group.

Seedhouse, D. (1986). *Health: the Foundations of Achievement*. Chichester, John Wiley.

Seeman, T.E. and Berkman, L.F. (1988). 'Structural characteristics of social networks and their relationship with social support in the elderly: who provides support?' *Social Science and Medicine*, 26: 737–49.

Seeman, T.E., Kaplan, G.A., Knudsen, L. *et al.* (1987). 'Social network ties and mortality among the elderly in the Alameda County study.' *American Journal of Epidemiology*, 126: 714–23.

Shanas, E., Townsend, P. and Wedderburn, D. *et al.* (1968). *Old People in Three Industrial Societies*. London, Routledge and Kegan Paul.

Shin, D.C. and Johnson, D.M. (1978). 'Avowed happiness as an overall assessment of the quality of life.' *Social Indicators Research*, 5: 475–92.

Silber, E. and Tippett, J. (1965). 'Self esteem: clinical assessment and measurement validation.' *Psychological Reports*, 16: 1017–71.

Sims, A.C.P. and Salmons, P.H. (1975). 'Severity of symptoms of psychiatric out-patients: use of the General Health Questionnaire in hospital and general practice patients.' *Psychological Medicine*, 5: 62–6.

Singer, E., Garfinkel, R., Cohen, S.M. *et al.* (1976). 'Mortality and mental health: evidence from the midtown Manhattan re-study.' *Social Science and Medicine*, 10: 517–21.

Skinner, D.E. and Yett, D.E. (1972). 'Debility index for long-term care patients' in Berg, R.L. (ed.). *Health Status Indexes*. Chicago, Hospital Research and Education Trust.

Slevin, M.L. (1984). 'Quality of life in cancer patients.' *Clinics in Oncology*, 371–90.

Slevin, M.L., Plant, H., Lynch, D. *et al.* (1988). 'Who should measure quality of life, the doctor or the patient?' *British Journal of Cancer*, 57: 109–12.

Smith, A. (1987). Qualms about qualys. *Lancet*, 1: 1134–6.

Smith, A.H.W., Ballinger, B.R. and Presley, A.S. (1981). 'The reliability and validity of two assessment scales for the elderly mentally handicapped.' *British Journal of Psychiatry*, 138: 15–16.

Smith, T.W. (1979). 'Happiness: time trends, seasonal variations, inter-survey differences and other mysteries.' *Social Psychology Quarterly*, 42: 18–30.

Snaith, R.P. (1987). 'The concepts of mild depression.' *British Journal of Psychiatry*, 150: 387–93.

Sokolovsky, J. (1986). 'Network methodologies in the study of ageing' in Keith, J. (ed.). *New Methods for Old Age Research*. Greenwood, Bergin and Garvey.

Spatz, K. and Johnson, F. (1973). 'Internal consistency of the Coopersmith Self Esteem Inventory.' *Educational and Psychological Measurements*, 33: 875–6.

Spector, W.D., Katz, S., Murphy, J.B. *et al.* (1987). 'The hierarchical relationship between activities of daily living and instrumental activities of daily living.' *Journal of Chronic Diseases*, 40: 481–9.

Spitzer, R.L., Burdock, E.I. and Hardesty, A.S. (1964). *Mental Status Schedule.* New York, Department of Psychiatry, College of Physicians and Surgeons, Columbia University and Biometrics Research Section, New York State Department of Mental Hygiene.

Spitzer, R.L., Endicott, J., Fliess, J.L. *et al.* (1970). 'Psychiatric status schedule: a technique for evaluating psychopathology and impairment in role functioning.' *Archives of General Psychiatry*, 23: 41–55.

Spitzer, R.L., Endicott, J. and Robins, E. (1978). 'Research Diagnostic Criteria: rationale and reliability.' *Archives of General Psychiatry*, 35: 773–82.

Spitzer, W.O., Dobson, A.J., Hall, J. *et al.* (1981). 'Measuring quality of life of cancer patients: a concise QL-index for use by physicians.' *Journal of Chronic Diseases*, 34: 585–97.

Springfield, V.A. (1976). *Perceived Health and Patient Role Propensity.* Washington, DC, Department of Commerce, National Technical Information Service.

Stehouwer, R.S. (1985). 'Beck Depression Inventory' in Keyser, D.J. and Sweetland, R.C. (eds). *Test Critiques*, vol. II. Kansas City, Missouri, Test Corporation of America.

Stewart, A.L., Greenfield, S., Hays, R.D. *et al.* (1989). 'Functional status and well-being of patients with chronic conditions: results from the medical outcomes study.' *Journal of the American Medical Association*, 262: 907–13.

Stewart, A. and Ware, J.E. (in press). Measuring behavioral functioning and well-being: The medical outcomes study approach.

Stewart, A.L., Hays, R.D. and Ware, J.E. (1988). 'The MOS Short-form General Health Survey. Reliability and validity in a patient population.' *Medical Care*, 26.: 724–35.

Stewart, A.L., Ware, J.E. and Brook, R.H. (1981). 'Advances in the measurement of functional status: construction of aggregate indexes.' *Medical Care*, 19: 473–88.

Stewart, A.L., Ware, J.E., Brook, R.H. *et al.* (1978). *Conceptualization and Measurement of Health for Adults in the Health Insurance Study*: vol. II: *Physical Health in Terms of Functioning.* Santa Monica, Rand Corporation: R-1987/2-HEW.

Stock, W.A. and Okun, M.A. (1982). 'The construct validity of life satisfaction among the elderly.' *Journal of Gerontology*, 37: 625–7.

Stokes, J.P. (1983). 'Predicting satisfaction with social support from social network structure.' *American Journal of Community Psychology*, 11: 141–52.

—— (1985). 'The relation of social network and individual difference variables to loneliness.' *Journal of Personality and Social Psychology*, 48: 981–90.

Stokes, J.P. and Wilson, D.G. (1984). 'The Inventory of Socially Supportive Behaviours: dimensionality, prediction and gender differences.' *American Journal of Community Psychology*, 12: 53–70.

Stones, M.L. and Kozma, A. (1980). 'Issues relating to the usage of conceptualizations of mental constructs employed by gerontologists.' *International Journal of Ageing and Human Development*, 11: 269–81.

Streiner, D.L. and Norman, G.R. (1989). *Health Measurement Scales: A Practical Guide to their Development and Use.* Oxford, Oxford University Press.

Stueve, A. and Lein, L. (1979). 'Problems in network analysis: the case of the missing person.' Paper presented at 32nd annual general meeting of the Gerontological Society.

Stull, D.E. (1987). 'Conceptualization and measurement of well-being: implications for policy evaluation' in Borgatta, E.F. and Montgomery, R.J.V. (eds). *Critical Issues in Ageing Policy.* Beverly Hills, Sage Publications.

Sullivan, C.F., Copeland, J.R.M., Dewey, M.E. *et al.* (1988). 'Benzodiazepine usage amongst the elderly: findings of the Liverpool community survey.' *International Journal of Geriatric Psychiatry*, 3: 289–92.

Tardy, C.H. (1985). 'Social support measurement.' *American Journal of Community Psychiatry*, 13: 187–202.

Tarnopolsky, A., Hand, D.J., McLean, E.K. *et al.* (1979). Validity and uses of a screening questionnaire (GHQ) in the community.' *British Journal of Psychiatry*, 134: 508–15.

Taylor, J. and Reitz, W. (1968). *The Three Faces of Self-esteem.* London, University of Western Ontario, Department of Psychology. Research Bulletin no. 80.

Teeling Smith, G. (1988). *Measuring Health: A Practical Approach.* Chichester, John Wiley.

Tennant, C. (1977). 'The General Health Questionnaire: a valid index of psychological impairment in Australian populations.' *Medical Journal of Australia*, 2: 392–4.

Thoits, P.A. (1982). 'Conceptual, methodological and theoretical problems in studying social support as a buffer against life stress.' *Journal of Health and Social Behaviour*, 23: 145–59.

Thomas, M.R. and Lyttle, D. (1980). 'Patient expectations about success of treatment and reported relief from low back pain.' *Journal of Psychosomatic Research*, 24: 297–301.

Thompson, C. (1984). *The Reliability of a Schedule for Assessing Dependency in the Elderly in Residential Care.* Manchester, University of Manchester. Working papers in applied social research, no. 2.

Thompson, P. and Blessed, G. (1987). 'Correlation between the 37-item Mental Test Score and abbreviated 10-item Mental Test Score by psychogeriatric day patients.' *British Journal of Psychiatry*, 151: 206–9.

Thompson, W. (1972). *Correlates of the Self Concept.* Nashville, Tennessee, Counselor Recordings and Tests.

Thuriaux, M.C. (1988). 'Health promotion and indicators for health for all in the European Region.' *Health Promotion*, 3: 89–99.

Toevs, C.D., Kaplan, R.M. and Atkins, C.J. (1984). 'The costs and effects of behavioral programs in chronic obstructive pulmonary disease.' *Medical Care*, 22: 1088–1100.

Tolsdorf, C.C. (1976). 'Social networks, support and coping: an exploratory study.' *Family Process*, 15: 407–17.

Toner, J., Gurland, B. and Teresi, J. (1988). 'Comparison of self-administered and rater-administered methods of assessing levels of severity of depression in elderly patients.' *Journal of Gerontology*, 43: 136–40.

Torrance, G.W. (1986). 'Measurement of health state utilities for economic appraisal.' *Journal of Health Economics*, 5: 1–30.

Townsend, P. (1962). *The Last Refuge.* London, Routledge and Kegan Paul.

—— (1979). *Poverty in the United Kingdom.* Harmondsworth, Pelican.

Trowbridge, N. (1970). 'Effects of socio-economic class on self-concept of children.' *Psychology in the Schools*, 7: 304–6.

Twining, T.C. and Allen, D.G. (1981). 'Disability factors among residents in old people's homes.' *Journal of Epidemiology and Community Health*, 36: 303–5.

Usui, W.M., Keil, T.J. and Durig, K.R. (1985). 'Socioeconomic comparisons and life satisfaction of elderly adults.' *Journal of Gerontology*, 40: 110–14.

Vacchiano, R.B. and Strauss, P.S. (1968). 'The construct validity of the Tennessee Self Concept Scale.' *Journal of Clinical Psychology*, 24: 323–6.

Valdenegro, J. and Barrera, M. (1983). 'Social support as a moderator of life stress: a longitudinal study using a multi-method analysis', paper presented at the meeting of the Western Psychological Association, San Francisco, California.

Vardon, V.M. and Blessed, G. (1986). 'Confusion ratings and abbreviated mental test performance: a comparison.' *Age and Ageing*, 15: 139–44.

Vaux, A. and Wood, J. (1985) 'Social support resources, behaviors and appraisals: a path analysis', paper presented at the meeting of the Midwestern Psychological Association, Chicago.

Vaux, A., Burda, P. and Stewart, D. (1986a). 'Orientation toward utilizing support resources.' *Journal of Community Psychology*, 14: 159–70.

Vaux, A., Phillips, J., Holly, L. *et al.* (1986b). *American Journal of Community Psychology*, 14: 195–219.

Vaux, A., Riedel, S. and Stewart, D. (1987). 'Modes of social support: the social support behaviours (SS-B) scale.' *American Journal of Community Psychology*, 15: 209–33.

Vetter, N. and Ford, D. (1989). 'Anxiety and depression scores in elderly fallers.' *International Journal of Geriatric Psychiatry*, 4: 159–63.

Vetter, N., Jones, D.A. and Victor, C.R. (1982). 'The importance of mental disabilities for the use of services by the elderly.' *Journal of Psychosomatic Research*, 26: 607–12.

Vetter, N., Smith, A., Sastry, D. and Tinker, G. (1989). *Day hospital – pilot study report*. Research Team for the Care of Elderly People, Department of Geriatrics, St. David's Hospital, Cardiff, S. Wales.

Vieweg, B.W. and Hedlund, J.L. (1983). 'The General Health Questionnaire: a comprehensive review.' *Journal of Operational Psychiatry*, 14: 74–81.

Vincent, J. (1968). 'An explanatory factor analysis relating to the construct validity of self concept labels.' *Educational and Psychological Measurement*, 28: 915–21.

Wade, D.T. and Collin, C. (1988). The Barthel ADL Index: a standard measure of physical disability. *International Disability Studies*, 10: 64–67.

Walker, K., Macbride, A. and Vachon, M.L.S. (1977). 'Social support networks and the crisis of bereavement.' *Social Science and Medicine*, 11: 34–41.

Walsh, J.A. (1984). 'Tennessee Self Concept Scale' in Keyser, D.J. and Sweetland, R.C. (eds). *Test Critiques*, vol. 1. Kansas City, Missouri, Test Corporation of America.

Wan, T.T.H. and Livieratos, B. (1977). 'A validation of the General Well-being Index: a two-stage multivariate approach, paper presented at American Public Health Association meeting, Washington DC.

Ward, R.A. (1977). 'The impact of subjective age and stigma on older persons.' *Journal of Gerontology*, 32: 227–32.

Ward, R.A., Sherman, S.R. and LaGory, M. (1984). 'Subjective network assessments and subjective well-being.' *Journal of Gerontology*, 39: 93–101.

Ware, J.E. (1984). 'Methodological considerations in the selection of health status assessment procedures' in Wenger, N.K., Mattson, M.E., Furberg, C.D. *et al.* (eds). *Assessment of Quality of Life in Clinical Trials of Cardiovascular Therapies.* New York, Le Jacq Publ. Co. Inc.

—— (1986). 'The assessment of health status' in Aiken, L.H. and Mechanic, D. (eds). *Applications of Social Science to Clinical Medicine and Health Policy.* New Brunswick, New Jersey, Rutgers University Press.

Ware, J.E. and Karmos, A.H. (1976). *Development and Validation of Scales to Measure Perceived Health and Patient Role Propensity,* vol. 2 of a final report. Carbondale, Illinois, Southern Illinois University School of Medicine, publication no. PB 288-331.

Ware, J.E. and Young, J. (1979). 'Issues in the conceptualization and measurement of value placed on health' in Mushkin, S.J. and Dunlop, D.W. (eds). *Health: what is it worth?* New York, Pergamon Press.

Ware, J.E., Brook, R.H., Davies-Avery, A. *et al.* (1980). *Conceptualization and Measurement of Health for Adults in the Health Insurance Study,* vol. 6, *Analysis of Relationships among Health Status Measures.* Santa Monica, CA, Rand Corporation: R1987/6-HEW.

Ware, J.E., Johnson, S.A., Davies-Avery, A. *et al.* (1979). *Conceptualization and Measurement of Health for Adults in the Health Insurance Study,* vol. III, *Mental Health.* Santa Monica, CA, Rand Corporation: R-1987/3-HEW.

Warr, P. (1978). 'A study of psychological well-being.' *British Journal of Psychology,* 69: 111-21.

Watson, E. and Evans, S. (1986). 'An example of cross-cultural measurement of psychological symptoms in post-partum mothers.' *Social Science and Medicine,* 23: 869-74.

Webb, E.J., Campbell, D.T., Schwartz, R.D. *et al.* (1966). *Unobtrusive Measures: Non-reactive Research in the Social Sciences.* Chicago, Rand McNally College Publishing.

Weckowicz, T., Muir, W. and Cropley, A. (1967). 'A factor analysis of the Beck Inventory of Depression.' *Journal of Consulting Psychology,* 31: 23-8.

Weiss, R.S. (1969). 'The fund of sociability.' *Transactions,* 6: 36.

—— (1973). *Loneliness: The Experience of Emotional and Social Isolation.* Cambridge, MA, MIT Press.

Wells, E. and Marwell, G. (1976). *Self Esteem.* Beverly Hills, Sage Publications.

Wells, K.B., Hays, R.D., Burnam, M.A., *et al.* (1989). Detection of depressive disorder for patients receiving pre-paid or fee for service care. Results from the Medical Outcomes Study. *Journal of the American Medical Association,* 262: 3298-3302.

Wells, K.B., Stewart, A., Hays, R.D. *et al.* (1989). 'The functioning and well-being of depressed patients: results from the medical outcomes study.' *Journal of the American Medical Association,* 262: 914-19.

Wenger, N.K., Mattson, M.E., Furberg, C.D. *et al.* (eds) (1984). *Assessment of Quality of Life in Clinical Trials of Cardiovascular Therapies.* USA, Le Lacq Pub. Inc.

Wentowski, G. (1982). 'Reciprocity and the coping strategies of older people: cultural dimensions of network building.' *Gerontologist,* 21: 600-9.

WHO (1958). *The First Ten Years. The Health Organization.* Geneva, World Health Organization.

—— (1980). *International Classification of Impairments, Disabilities and Handicaps.* Geneva, World Health Organization.

—— (1982). *Basic Documents.* (32nd edition). Geneva, World Health Organization.

—— (1985). *Targets for Health for All by the Year 2000.* Copenhagen, World Health Organization. Regional Office for Europe.

Wiest, W.M. (1965). 'A qualitative extension of Heider's theory of cognitive balance applied to interpersonal perception and self esteem.' *Psychological Monographs: General and Applied*, 79: 1–20.

Wilkin, D. (1987). 'Conceptual problems in dependency research.' *Social Science and Medicine*, 24: 867–73.

Wilkin, D. and Jolley, D.J. (1979). *Behavioural Problems among Old People in Geriatric Wards, Psychogeriatric Wards and Residential Homes, 1976–78.* Research Report no. 1, Research Section, Psychiatric Unit, University Hospital of South Manchester.

Wilkin, D. and Thompson, C. (1989). *User's Guide to Dependency Measures for Elderly People.* Sheffield Social Services Monographs: Research in Practice. University of Sheffield, Joint Unit for Social Services Research.

Wilkin, D., Mashiah, T. and Jolley, D.J. (1978). 'Changes in behavioural characteristics of elderly populations of local authority homes and long stay hospital wards, 1976–77.' *British Medical Journal*, 2: 1274–6.

Willcocks, D., Peace, S. and Kellaher, L. (1987). *Private Lives in Public Places.* London, Tavistock Press.

Williams, J.M.G. (1984). *The Psychology of Depression.* Beckenham, Croom Helm.

Williams, P. (1987). 'Depressive thinking in general practice patients' in Freeling, P., Downey, L.J. and Malkin, J.C. (eds). *The Presentation of Depression: Current Approaches.* Royal College of General Practitioners, Occasional Paper, 36: 17–20.

Williams, R.G.A., Johnston, M., Willis, M. *et al.* (1976). 'Disability: a model and measurement technique.' *British Journal of Preventive and Social Medicine*, 30: 71–8.

Williams, S.J. and Bury, M.J. (1989). 'Impairment, disability and handicap in chronic respiratory illness.' *Social Science and Medicine*, 29: 609–16.

Wilson, L.A. and Brass, W. (1973). 'Brief assessment of the mental state in geriatric domiciliary practice: the usefulness of the mental status questionnaire.' *Age and Ageing*, 2: 92–101.

Wilson, L.A., Roy, S.K. and Bursill, A.E. (1973). 'The reliability of the mental status questionnaire in geriatric practice'. (Unpublished, cited in Wilson and Brass.)

Wilson Barnett, J. (1981). 'Assessment of recovery: with special reference to a study with post-operative cardiac patients.' *Journal of Advanced Nursing*, 6: 435–45.

Wing, J.K., Cooper, J.E. and Sartorius, N. (1974). *The Measurement and Classification of Psychiatric Symptoms: An Instruction Manual for the PSE and catego program.* Cambridge, Cambridge University Press.

Wood, V., Wylie, M.L. and Scheafor, B. (1969). 'An analysis of a short self-report measure of life satisfaction: correlation with rater judgements.' *Journal of Gerontology*, 24: 465–9.

Wylie, C.M. and White, B.K. (1964). 'A measure of disability'. *Archives of Environmental Health*, 8: 834–9.

Wylie, M.L. (1970). 'Life satisfaction as a program impact criterion.' *Journal of Gerontology*, 25: 36–40.

Wylie, R.C. (1974). *The Self Concept*. Lincoln, Nebraska, University of Nebraska Press.

Zigmond, A.S. and Snaith, R.P. (1983). 'The Hospital Anxiety and Depression Scale.' *Acta Psychiatrica Scandinavica*, 67: 361–70.

Ziller, R., Hagey, J., Smith, M.D. *et al.* (1969). 'Self-esteem: a social construct.' *Journal of Consulting and Clinical Psychology*, 33: 84–95.

Zung, W.W.K. (1965). 'A self-rating depression scale.' *Archives of General Psychiatry*, 12: 63–70.

—— (1967). 'Depression in the normal aged.' *Psychosomatics*, 8: 287–92.

Zung, W.W.K., Richards, C.B. and Short, M.J. (1965). 'Self rating depression scale in an out-patient clinic: further validation of the SDS.' *Archives of General Psychiatry*, 13: 508–15.